I0027042

The Birthing Goddess

The Birthing Goddess

Reclaiming the Legacy of Natural, Pain-Free Childbirth

LAILA VALERE

Waterside Productions

Copyright © 2020 by Laila Valere

All rights reserved. This book or any portion thereof may not be reproduced or used in any manner whatsoever without the express written permission of the publisher except for the use of brief quotations in articles and book reviews.

Cover picture of Angelique Valere-Beaubrun by Amada Egan

Cover design by Ken Fraser

Illustrations by Amada Egan and Angelique Valere-Beaubrun

Printed in the United States of America

First Printing, 2020

ISBN-13: 978-1-949001-32-7 print edition
ISBN-13: 978-1-949001-33-4 ebook edition

Waterside Productions
2055 Oxford Ave
Cardiff, CA 92007
www.waterside.com

Dedication

*I dedicate this book to
my mother Zanimoon Sultan-Khan, the kindest and most forgiving
person I know who still inspires me to be the best that I can be,
and to
all my marvelous grandchildren who give me much hope for the
future: Aliena, Tiffany, Zachary, Logan, Zan, Joshua, Luc, Jean, Leo
and ....*

"This wonderful, timely book, THE BIRTHING GODDESS, reminds us that birthing is a Spiritual Event. For over 70 years I have been involved with the birthing of babies. Unfortunately, over time, this miraculous event has been reduced to a medical event. We must shift our concept from the medical aspect of pregnancy as a "diagnosis" to the spiritual, emotional, and physical process of birthing a baby. It is time we give the power back to the mother. We recognize that we must place the power and responsibility for birthing back in the hands of mothers with the understanding that doctors and midwives don't deliver babies, women do. This compelling book brings back the sacredness of the birthing process and the reverence for the new life that has been created."

—Dr. Gladys Taylor McGarey, MD, MD (H)

Acknowledgements - Expression of Gratitude

Thank you, thank you, thank you God for giving me the inspiration, courage, ability and all the assistance I needed to write this book. You have again helped me to appreciate the true meaning of being a co-creator.

I am profoundly grateful to be a Birthing Goddess.

I give thanks to all the Heavenly angels for their spiritual support and guidance – especially to my mother Zanimoon Sultan-Khan and to my son Emile Amral Laurence Valere.

My Earth angels have helped me in innumerable ways: My husband and companion-in-life, Michael, who gives me invaluable advice, space, and support to fulfill my goals; my first-born son, Marcus ,who was the first member of my family to read the entire manuscript and share his comments with me; my 2 precious daughters – true earth angels – Angelique and Athena who are now my best friends, giving me consistent, on-going emotional support and encouragement as well as deciphering, typing, and formatting most of my handwritten script; my brother Kameal who read and edited the very first chapter I wrote and gave me valuable suggestions on how to proceed; my sister Fareeda and brother Shafeek who are always there for me in all my ups and downs; my 2 daughters-in-law Juliette and Renata for their interest and also their assistance in typing the manuscript; my lifetime cherished and loyal friend Marilyn who helped to get me unstuck from my debilitating grief after the loss of my son Emile, restored my faith in my ability to complete this book and patiently edited my rough draft; my new friend

Yiara whose enthusiasm, valuable feedback, and typing skills helped me to make progress; Julia Gabell for her editorial expertise; Dr. Harry Ramnarine for taking time from his extremely busy schedule to read my manuscript and give me insightful feedback; my spiritual sisters (26 years of regular group meditation) for all their physical, mental, emotional and spiritual support as we journey together on the spiritual path; all the researchers and authors who have contributed to my knowledge and stirred my passion on this subject, in particular: Dr. Grantly Dick-Read, Deepak Chopra, and Marie Mongan; many, many magnificent human beings such as Oprah Winfrey, Marianne Williamson, Dr. Wayne Dyer, Eckhart Tolle, Sarah Ban Breathnach, Thich Nhat Hanh, Louise Hay, and Shakti Gawain for their inspirational messages that kept me going on the right track; and more recently, William Gladstone and Josh Freel of Waterside Productions for their knowledgeable and wise guidance in making my dream of publishing *The Birthing Goddess* a reality.

In a more universal way, every human being contributed to the creative process of producing *The Birthing Goddess*. The success of this book is the joint achievement of all.

Thank you everyone and May God bless us all.

Contents

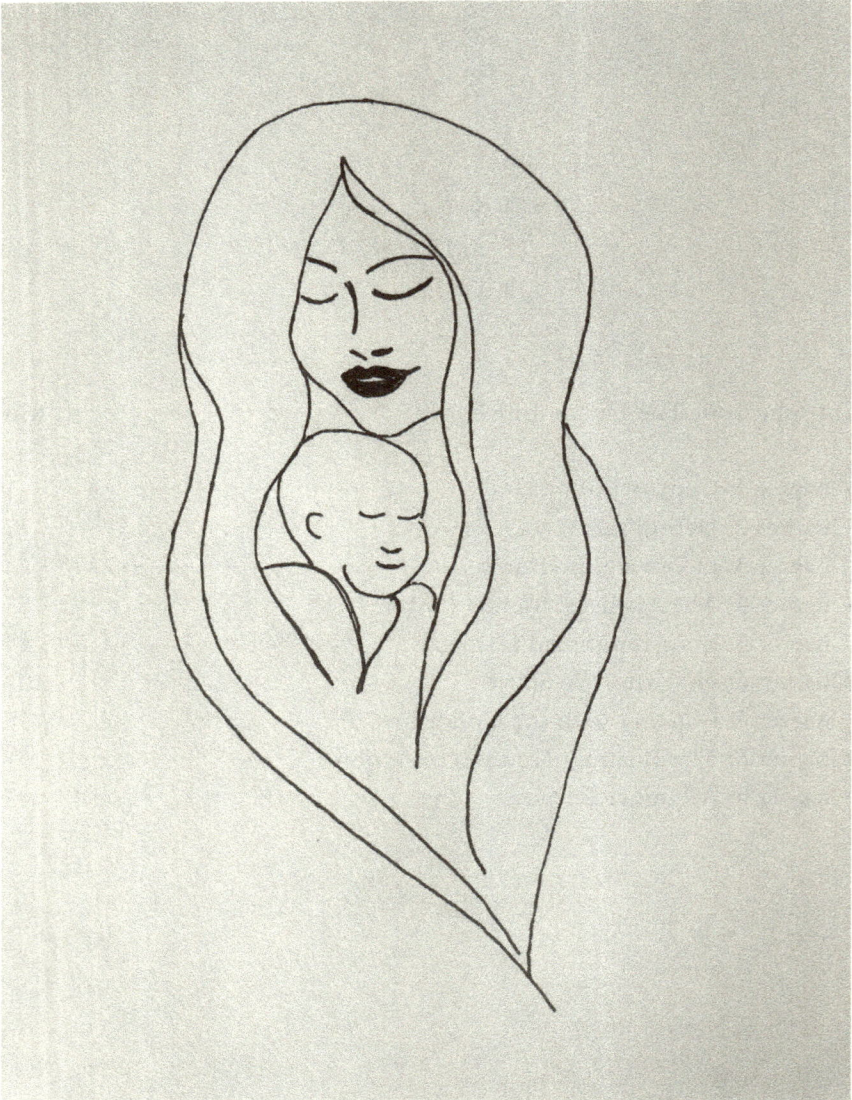

Introduction
My Credo

I firmly believe that all women are Birthing Goddesses.

I firmly believe that mothering and birthing begin from conception and continue throughout life.

I firmly believe that birthing was not meant to be a painful ordeal, but a natural, pain free, uplifting spiritual experience.

I firmly believe that Birthing Goddesses, during their pregnancies, can lay a strong foundation of peace and love in their children.

I firmly believe that Birthing Goddesses hold the power to bring peace to our world.

I firmly believe that all women can regain their Divine legacy as Birthing Goddesses.

I firmly believe that our Divine Creator will guide and help us all to be authentic human beings.

These beliefs resonate from my soul and motivate me to share my beliefs with others.

Introduction ~ The Divine Infusion

The spirit of the Birthing Goddess is in every woman waiting to be birthed.

As a Birthing Goddess you can experience the true beauty and joyfulness of birthing naturally and normally without pain. I have been privileged to enjoy such a birthing experience, and I wish to share what I did so that you, too, can have a superior birthing experience.

This structured holistic training program will serve to develop your God-given capabilities to the point where you can reclaim your power and true identity as a Birthing Goddess. As a Birthing Goddess you are empowered to:

- Enjoy a healthy, happy pregnancy and a safe, comfortable, fulfilling birthing
- Sow the seeds of peace and love into the children you birth as well as into all your relationships
- Release fear and negativity from your psyche
- Take greater control of your life and make informed, wiser choices
- Live your life with the confidence, serenity, and joyfulness of an enlightened being
- Be the best you can be
- Help others to develop their own potential

- Serve all of humanity and light up the world
- Surrender yourself to Divine Power

The information and training exercises in this book will be equally beneficial for men who also wish to more fully develop their own potential in a holistic, balanced manner.

This program can empower men to:

- Enjoy greater fulfillment from actively participating in the total process of co-creating new life throughout pregnancy, birthing, and parenting
- Achieve greater success in all their endeavors
- Express themselves as more authentic human beings
- Work conscientiously to promote and maintain peace and harmony in our world.

This book has been incubating in my mind and heart from the time of the birth of my youngest child, Athena. Since then I have collected information the universe has presented to me from many sources:

- My training and practice in counseling psychology, education, neuro-linguistic programming (NLP), hypnotherapy, mind mapping, breath-work, leadership development, yoga, chi gong, quantum touch healing, and meditation
- Extensive reading and research on this and related topics
- While assisting young pregnant women to develop a more positive attitude toward childbirth
- My own experiences of birthing four children
- The Collective Consciousness of the Universe.

I have drawn from these sources — organizing, combining, synthesizing and allowing the whole Gestalt to develop from its many parts. The result is this comprehensive, holistic program which involves the preparation of your total being to achieve a harmonious balance of body, mind, and spirit.

Many books have been dedicated to making childbirth a more comfortable experience and utilizing more natural procedures. I am pleased to be acting in unison with like-minded people. We all draw from each other and support each other as we move ahead to promote more positive experiences in an enlightened world.

Since this is a holistic approach, you will find that several of the techniques suggested here are similar to those offered in other childbirth training programs. These techniques will be incorporated into the relevant areas in this holistic program. You will also find powerful exercises that integrate physical, mental, emotional, and spiritual components into unified and amazingly effective training techniques.

The spiritual component is emphasized as fundamental, since it is our Divine Creator Who is ultimately responsible for the creation of all life. I believe that pregnancy and birthing is essentially *a spiritual event* which utilizes our physical, mental, emotional, and spiritual resources – all aspects of our human nature.

How To Use This Book Well

"What we are is God's gift to us, what we make of ourselves is our gift to God".

Anonymous

By taking a holistic approach to your preparation for pregnancy and birthing you are committing all your personal resources (physical, mental, emotional, and spiritual) to work towards achieving your goal of being a true Birthing Goddess. This is a dynamic process that involves activating, taking control of, and developing each of these resources in a balanced manner.

Each chapter in this book focuses on a specific area while maintaining its holistic framework.

Chapter 1: **Getting It Right** describes some of my own experiences during pregnancy and childbirth. It details my efforts at 'getting it right'. My hope is that these insights can inspire you to get it right for you and your baby.

Chapter 2: **Debriefing Myths** discusses some of the major misconceptions about birthing. In this chapter I also address the existing negative programming and systems that continue to keep us chained down to being victims of fear and pain and less than our Divine selves. You will have a better chance of achieving success if you can first dispel these myths and cleanse yourself of negative programming.

Chapter 3: **Honoring Your Body** focuses on your physical development. Co-creating a new life is a nine-month process. This gives adequate time to nurture and strengthen your body and improve your general fitness and health before birthing. Body changes take place gradually, allowing you time to adjust – another blessing from nature. In this chapter, I address the fundamental aspects of your physical training: conscious breath work, rest and relaxation, exercise, nutrition and body care. They are all important. You will find that most of these can easily fit into your daily routine. Like the weight lifter whose goal is to bench press 400 pounds, or the marathon runner whose goal is to complete the course in record time, you too must be motivated to train consistently. Your goal is deserving of the highest effort.

A word of caution here: Before you engage in any physical development program, it is always wise to get the sanction from your doctor or health-care provider. Please do so. Begin your program slowly and gently. Gradually increase the time and effort spent on each area as your proficiency and needs develop. And do remember to enjoy your training. Consider it your fun time!

Chapter 4: **The Magic of Mental Power** concentrates on your mental preparation. One of the biggest problems facing expectant mothers today is the lack of thorough and structured mental preparation. There are many prenatal training programs that focus mainly on physical preparation with only limited aspects of mental and emotional input. Birthing is only partly about physical fitness. To think otherwise is to trivialize the value of our mental power. What I offer in this chapter is a more comprehensive, structured and effective mental training program that will specifically prepare you to fully keep your focus and control during your birthing experience. These techniques and exercises will also incorporate physical, emotional, and spiritual components that strengthen their effectiveness. When you and your partner practice these exercises, your own mental power will increase greatly so that you will also be able to be more productive in all areas of your life.

This mental training program is a down-to-earth approach to applying basic psychological principles to the birthing performance. Yes, birthing is a *performance* and probably one of the greatest performances of your life. The mental training techniques outlined here have been tried and tested by world-class professional performers in many areas, especially in the field of sports where physical, mental and emotional strength and balance are necessary for superior performance – just as in birthing.

This mental program will help you to:

- Improve your ability to concentrate and focus
- Program your own mind and control your thoughts
- Develop and utilize your imagery skills
- Increase your self confidence
- Mentally relax when necessary
- Strengthen your motivation to succeed
- Utilize self hypnosis for pain free birthing

Chapter 5: *Your Emotional Garden* focuses on your emotional preparation. Scientific research and empirical evidence have shown that a pregnant woman's emotions are transmitted to her fetus and can affect the baby's growth and overall development in a positive or negative way. Negative emotions such as fear, anger, excessive stress, and depression all have a negative effect on the unborn baby with possible far-reaching implications after birth. Positive emotions such as peace, love, joyfulness, and contentment all have a positive effect on the baby. This chapter provides effective techniques and strategies for eliminating and managing negative emotions as well as ways to foster and maintain positive emotions and attitudes during pregnancy, birthing, and motherhood. Here you will also find activities which offer you an opportunity for self-reflection and greater self-awareness.

Chapter 6: *Nuturing the Spirit* stresses the importance of strengthening your spirituality. As a pregnant Birthing Goddess you manifest your spiritual connection and your Divine role in procreation. You and your partner join with the Divine to co-create new members of the human race. The strength of this partnership determines to a great degree the quality of your experience as a Birthing Goddess. I offer suggestions to strengthen your prayer power as well as to deepen your meditation. I also include the script of a guided meditation for you to use in your practice sessions.

Chapter 7: *Dancing with the Goddess* points out that pregnancy, birthing, and parenting is a family affair involving father, partner, family members, friends and health caregivers – all vital members of the co-creation team. This chapter focuses on the roles, responsibilities, and preparation of fathers and partners so that they can actively participate in the awesome process of co-creating new life.

Chapter 8: *The Birthing Goddess in Action* focuses on pulling it all together and putting it into action. For your convenience you will find a holistic development checklist and a suggested format to help you to organize your own Weekly Action Plan. Then the focus turns to planning for the actual birthing. I include worksheets for a "What If?" planner and another for you to list roles and expectations for the members of your birthing team. There is also a descriptive projection of what the birthing experience can be for you which will be helpful when you are practicing your mental rehearsal exercises.

Chapter 9: *A Higher Purpose* calls upon Birthing Goddesses and their partners to commit themselves to promoting peace and goodwill in our world. It shows how this honorable effort begins with personal development, birthing, parenting and living with integrity. I then end with a Benediction, as a gift from one Birthing Goddess to another Birthing Goddess.

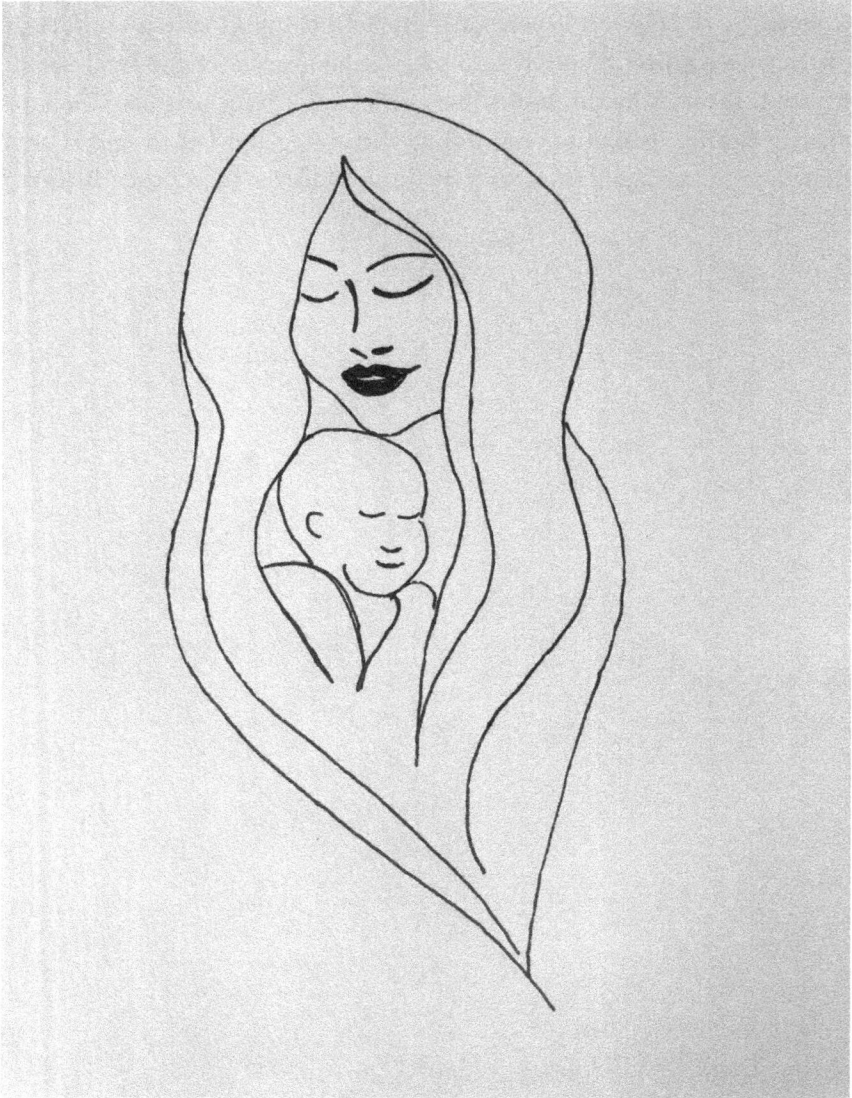

Chapter 1
Getting It Right

My Experience

"Congratulations! You're pregnant!"

"Uh???!! Impossible. It can't be."

Mike and I look at each other in bewilderment and shock.

"Are you sure?"

"Yes, of course. You are 2 ½ – 3 months pregnant."

"But that can't be. I have already completed menopause."

"You are 45 years old?" the doctor asked, obviously expecting me to confirm what was recorded in my chart.

"No, I am 35 years old," I responded mechanically.

"There seems to be a 10 year discrepancy here," remarked the young doctor looking closely at my chart. *"How old did you say you were?"*

Feeling a little foolish, I offered an explanation. *"Right now, I still feel and act as I did 10 years ago – that's why I think 35!*

"Well, that explains your pregnancy!" he said. *"When was your last period?"*

"Period? I stopped that long ago—about two years now. I have been through menopause already. No, no! There must be some mistake. I don't feel pregnant—no morning sickness, Nothing."

"Have you noticed any other signs?" asked the doctor.

I thought for a while. I had noticed some increased size in my mid section, so I had been doing yoga exercises and using a soap and cream treatment to remove the cellulite buildup on my waist and stomach. Angelique, my daughter, would help me to apply it and then scrub it on when I took my shower each day. I remember her recently commenting, *"Mom, I don't think that this is working; your stomach is getting bigger."*

I responded reluctantly to the doctor's question. *"Yes, my breasts do feel very tender and I have noticed increased size in my mid section."*

As the initial shock of this news wore off and the realization gradually set in, I felt nausea rising up in me, and I rushed out of the office into the washroom for my first bout of 'morning sickness.'

I returned to the doctor's office with tears flowing down my face and listened as Mike and the doctor discussed my options. I heard the doctor say:

- Having a baby at my age would put me and the baby in the 'high risk' category,
- One in four babies could present trisomy of chromosome 21, also known as Down Syndrome,
- Because of these factors he did not think that it would be wise to continue with the pregnancy and that I could safely terminate the pregnancy before it reached 4 months,
- If I chose to have the baby, he (the doctor) would recommend that I go to other more experienced doctors since he had never delivered a baby from a person as old as I was.

Mike and I walked out of the office in dead silence, each of us struggling with our own emotions. Then Mike started singing 'One day at a time, sweet Jesus'. I looked at him and had to smile. He can't carry a tune to save his life, but he was trying to cope with the enormity of this challenging and frightening situation in which we found ourselves.

'One day at a time sweet, Jesus' was to become my daily prayer. I cried all the way home.

My name is Laila.

I am married to Michael (Mike) and we have three children: Marcus, 16; Emile, 14; and Angelique (Ange), 12. I am 45 years old—yes, 45 years old and I had already completed menopause.

This is my pregnancy story.

The next few weeks were extremely turbulent. Michael felt strongly that I should terminate the pregnancy. And I felt that I couldn't … so we had long discussions, heated arguments, and fierce quarrels. He reiterated over and over all the doctor's recommendations, since they came from a knowledgeable and respected expert. Mike just couldn't understand why I wouldn't accept them … and so he added his own rationale:

1. We couldn't afford the cost of having a baby since we did not have maternity coverage.
2. At this point in our lives it would mean that we would have to change our lifestyle and life plans. We would have to invest time and effort in bringing up another child, and I might not be able to complete my Masters or Doctorate degrees.
3. Financially, a baby would be a huge strain on us – especially now that his business was not going too well.
4. Having recently moved from Trinidad to Florida, I would not have any help to look after a baby, so we might have to go back to Trinidad.
5. This situation would be a thousand times worse if the baby had Down Syndrome.
6. We already had three healthy children who we enjoyed and who would need our attention and financial support for their education.
7. We would be asking for trouble and we would be greedy, selfish, and stupid (meaning I would be) to want to continue with this pregnancy knowing all of the above.

He even got members of my family to support his position and to seek to influence me. Yes, his were powerful, convincing, and logical arguments. I concede that!

But my stance really had nothing to do with those factors.

I just could not bring myself to terminate this pregnancy. There was something deep inside of me that said, *"No, don't do that."*

What was it?

It was not because I was a 'goody, goody' or because I had strong religious beliefs or moralistic conviction. I had already had to terminate one pregnancy earlier in my marriage. I cannot remember clearly the exact circumstances or reasons why, except that my doctor had recommended it. I remember going to a nursing home/clinic and having it done there. The experience was comfortable and I had felt relieved when it was over.

After that, I had one more pregnancy which ended up as a miscarriage, and I was very emotionally upset about that. It was a girl and I really wanted another daughter so that Angelique could have a sister. Since that time we had been trying to have another child so we had not used any contraceptives. But I was not able to conceive again. I used to get 'babyitis' (longing to have and care for a baby) whenever I saw another baby. I looked forward to getting pregnant again – I remember being extremely happy and alive when I was pregnant. During those times I felt fulfilled and blessed.

I used to wonder why I didn't conceive again even though the gynecologist had said that there was nothing amiss. As years passed, I accepted my lot but continued to get occasional 'babyitis'.

I experienced early menopause and was no longer menstruating or having hot flashes or other discomforts. Menopause was over.

By that time, we had all moved to Florida where Mike was relocated on his job. I saw this as an opportunity for me to return to university, so I was very happy to make that move.

Our three children were no longer babies, and I felt I would have time to get my doctorate. I love learning––exams excite me–and I have always done well in school. So here I was, happily going for my Masters in Counseling Psychology, getting straight A's in all my courses, and feeling great.

The children were also doing well, and Mike was busy with his business. We had made good friends, and everything in our lives was comfortable and in place; so comfortable that my waist was getting bigger and my clothes were getting tighter. Mike felt it was my sedentary lifestyle– too much sitting and studying. So I started practicing yoga, playing tennis, and walking regularly. In addition I started using a cellulite soap/cream regimen to remove unsightly fat and cellulite deposits around my stomach.

Despite the extra weight, I was feeling in the pink of health and full of energy.

Mike decided at this point to take out another life insurance policy making it necessary for both of us to have full medical examinations. No problem. But the strangest thing happened after I had my physical examination by the doctor. The doctor then said that he was also going to do a pregnancy test on me.

I laughed and said to him, "You will be wasting your time and my money".

But he did it anyway. I left the office and went my merry way, not in the least bit concerned about the results of the pregnancy test.

A few days later, we got a call from the doctor requesting that Michael and I both come in to see him together. I thought that perhaps it had to do with Mike's high cholesterol or something similar. But instead we received the totally unexpected and shocking news that I was very pregnant.

What should we do?

Actually, that decision was up to me! The power to say "yes" or "no" was really in my hands. That was a frightening responsibility.

I wanted this child with all my heart and soul and mind and spirit.

I was not going to terminate this pregnancy, even though the odds seemed against me. I felt in my heart that I was being given another chance to have a baby girl and another opportunity to enjoy a wonderful pregnancy and to get it really right.

I knew that Mike would be very angry with me for the risk that I would be taking. Mike couldn't and wouldn't force me to terminate the pregnancy, but he certainly reacted strongly against my decision. He even took my decision personally, claiming that I did not respect his judgment and his feelings. He detached himself from me and withdrew his warmth and affection.

Our interactions became cold and polite for the next few months and we merely went through the motions of doing what was necessary.

This was the loneliest time of my life. But I was not alone. Our three children were as excited as I was about the growing baby and supported me fully. I remember well one of my doubtful moments. I was wondering aloud what would happen if something happened to me, and I couldn't look after the proper growth of this child. They all three promised that they would take responsibility for the nurturing and care of the baby. This warmed by heart and comforted me.

This was also the time of my life in which I grew spiritually strong. I prayed throughout the day; I begged God to help me; I bargained with Him. I promised Him that if he allowed me to have a safe delivery and a healthy, normal baby, I would in turn be the best person I could be and would always trust in Him and His guidance. I would devote my life to Him. I was negotiating with God!!!

"One day at a time, sweet Jesus, that's all I'm asking of you." I listened to that song by Christy Lane every day. It became my theme song. It rang in my ear.

I spent much time reflecting on God's influence in my life, recognizing and acknowledging more fully His presence and the many miracles that He had bestowed on me, on my family and friends. I drew inspiration from these experiences and especially from my own mother's strength, courage, tenacity, and unwavering faith even in the most trying situations.

I sat in meditation regularly every day, allowing my heart to convey my message to God. I found time to meditate both in the morning and in the evening. My meditation deepened and I often felt God's abiding presence within me. I began to learn the true meaning of surrendering to God as I allowed myself to receive and benefit from His Divine Guidance.

I continued my University course of studies in psychology. My course work became more meaningful and I experienced many "Aha!"

moments intellectually, spiritually, and emotionally. I realized that if I were to become a good psychologist, I must first apply these psychological concepts to myself. I realized that this whole experience was part of a Divine plan for me, designed to prepare me to take action on something I felt strongly about: birthing naturally and without pain, the way I believe God intended childbirth to be.

I embarked on a training program for my own Olympic performance, the birthing of my baby. At this point I took full ownership and responsibility for my baby, my gift from God, and I intended to work with God (and anyone he sent to help me) on this as a spiritual endeavor. I was determined to get it right this time.

I was not totally happy with the birthing experiences I had with my first three children. First of all, the deliveries took place in medical clinics housing sick persons. I did not consider myself sick. In fact, I was an extremely healthy woman engaged in a very healthy activity! The worst part for me was in the delivery rooms. I found them cold, sterile, unwelcoming, and downright intimidating. Was this where I must welcome my baby into this world? My legs were placed in stirrups. For whose convenience? Certainly not mine. How could I push effectively in such an awkward and disempowering position? I really hated those stirrups. They reminded me of the contraptions used in ancient times when preparing people for torture. I felt as if I were being asked to catch a ball with my hands tied behind my back.

I had attended prenatal natural birthing classes before having my first three children and I understood intellectually what takes place in the birthing process, but that helped me little to manage the serious and intense pain I felt during delivery. It was indeed torture at times. Was it really meant to be like that? I found it hard to believe that God who created women with the capacity to give birth intended the process to be so painful. Something went wrong there, and I wished it could be put right for me and every other birthing woman. Should my baby be held upside down by his leg and be slapped on his bottom to make him cry? A welcome of physical violence? There must be another gentler, more loving way to birth my baby.

Now, I was a little bit older, somewhat wiser, and being at university I had access to more up-to-date information. I researched and explored all the accepted and available books and programs for natural childbirth. Many of them validated my thinking, especially *childbirth without fear* written by Dr Grantly Dick-Read.

I became more determined than ever to have this baby naturally and without pain. I was convinced that, if God made woman and graced her with the ability to conceive and bring forth new life, then birthing was a normal and natural process. It was definitely not a medical problem automatically needing hospitalization, though I would utilize a doctor's help in monitoring the physical aspects of my pregnancy. After all, I admitted, doctors were also God's children, even though some of them behaved as if they themselves had the authority of God.

After much investigation, I found a group of four doctors who were willing to take my 'high risk' case, although they were skeptical about my wanting to have this baby naturally. My gut feeling was that they accepted me as their patient only because I was increasing their revenue. They didn't really show any caring. I was just another number on their books. They went through their required procedures and so did I.

I began exercising regularly to strengthen myself physically. I did most of my studying and reading while squatting with my back against a wall. I continued my yoga and attended childbirth education classes. Michael reluctantly accompanied me to those classes, even though he didn't see the need for him to participate in them. I really appreciated his efforts.

I ate the 'right' foods sensibly and, oh yes; I stopped smoking my one cigarette a day. I was not going to contaminate my baby in any way. Mike decided to stop smoking also. I guess he thought it was the right time to do so. With great effort and full support from our children, we both succeeded in breaking that addictive and harmful habit.

I practiced conscious breathing exercises and a form of progressive relaxation to give me more control over my muscles with focus on the pelvic area. I walked every day. The physical part of my training was consistent and progressed smoothly.

Spiritually, I was growing stronger and that refueled my spirit. I felt I was becoming more and more connected to God, and I knew that it was His grace that was helping me in every way, especially with my emotional needs.

Yet, there were times I struggled to manage my anxieties. I remember waiting for the results of the amniocentesis tests. I tried not to think of the worse-case scenario. The doctor had said that in older mothers statistics show that one in four babies is born with Down Syndrome. That thought was hard to get out of my head.

If the test showed that my baby was defective in any way, what would I do? I tried to make a Plan A and Plan B, but I shuddered at the thought every time. The implications were far too scary for me, so I kept putting those plans on hold.

So I prayed harder and harder and begged God to spare us that agonizing future. My anxiety would eventually subside as I surrendered more and more to God's will. I had to make an ongoing conscious effort every waking hour to keep my thoughts positive and to trust in God's love and mercy.

I practiced mental exercises to discipline my mind and to help me to keep my focus. I also started strengthening my visualization of holding in my arms a healthy, smiling baby. Several times a day I would breathe deeply, mentally visualize the growing fetus, fill myself with the purest love, and consciously transmit it to my baby. I saw these loving energies in translucent color as in a rainbow penetrating and flowing throughout my womb, embracing and caressing my baby with love and light until my baby was smiling with delight. I totally enjoyed this activity. It lifted my spirit. These efforts helped me to wait patiently and sometimes not so patiently for the result of the amniocentesis.

Then I received the news. I was lying in bed reading and Ange was lying next to me. The phone rang. I intuitively knew that this was what I was waiting for. I picked up the phone and heard that my baby was normal and healthy. I couldn't reply. I closed my eyes, became silent and still. This was confirmation that I had made the right choice. I could hear my inner voice repeating "Thank you, God; thank you, God; thank you,

God" until every cell of my body was resonating with thanks. I caressed my stomach and I sensed that my baby, too, was smiling with gratitude.

Tears were flowing down my face and Ange was shaking me and asking, "Mom, what is happening?"

I whispered quietly, "The baby is normal."

The voice on the other end of the phone was repeating, "Hello, hello! Are you there?"

Ange prompted me in the background, "Ask if it is a boy or girl."

"Yes, yes," I stuttered. "Thank you for calling–my baby is normal. Thank you."

"Do you want to know the gender?" the speaker asked.

"Yes, I do."

"Well, it's a girl."

"A girl! A girl!" I exclaimed. "Thank you."

Ange started jumping up and down on the bed, dancing and shouting, "It's a girl! It's a girl!"

I put down the phone and Ange and I hugged each other and then danced a jig around the room singing cheerfully "It's a girl and she is normal!" Wow!

I will never forget that feeling. It was the highest of highs. I was an Olympic winner; I had won the lottery. *"God, you are the best. Thank you! Thank you! Thank you!"* Total joyfulness.

We shared the great news with the family. Everyone was relieved and happy – especially Michael.

Now that I had received confirmation that my baby was normal, I became even more convinced that I was being given the opportunity to enjoy another pregnancy and to get the birthing right this time – a safe, natural, pain free and enjoyable delivery. This was the opportunity to use my God-given ability to be truly a Birthing Goddess. I became more strongly motivated and committed to achieving that goal.

The rest of the pregnancy flowed easily: regular exercise, a balanced nutritious diet, longer meditations, positive thoughts, beautiful, stronger visualizations and mental rehearsals of the birthing, and constructive planning for the arrival.

I started self-hypnosis training to strengthen my mental powers to help me gain greater control during the actual birthing stage. I also wanted to access a deeper level of consciousness where most discomfort would be eliminated. I had read a great deal about self-hypnosis and realized that it would also enhance and deepen my meditation. It certainly did.

The combination of self hypnosis and spiritual meditation aligned my body, mind, and spirit so that I was able to experience profound peace and relaxation at more beneficial levels of consciousness. I made sure that I found the time to practice my hypno-meditation at least once a day (most times twice a day for 20-30 minutes). It took a lot of careful juggling of study time, family time, and household duties, but I did it.

I felt myself getting stronger and stronger physically, mentally, emotionally, and spiritually. I was really enjoying the pregnancy. Michael himself was looking forward to the birth and showing more interest in me and in the process. I really needed and appreciated his support. That also made me feel a whole lot better.

I spoke to my baby often, sending loving messages to her telepathically. I played Schubert's serenade on the piano as well as other classical and lyrical music for her every day. I sang to her. I even shared with her all that I was learning at University, taking the time to explain complex information over and over until it became clearer to me. We were studying together. I engaged her as my partner in both my studies and her birthing. We were enjoying both activities and having fun too. I remember during one of my exams I couldn't recall the correct answer and I asked her to help me out and the answer promptly came to me. Did she respond to my call? I wonder. In the end, I made all A's in my final exam and completed my Masters with a 4.0 grade point average. Was there any connection? Did she really help me through it? Something to consider? I think so.

On reflection, I do believe that I received all the help I needed throughout this experience. I feel only gratitude to my immediate family, my friends, the Universe, and my Divine Creator for the support I received in whatever form it came.

The last stage of my pregnancy was totally enjoyable and fulfilling for me.

I partied, entertained and participated fully in the Christmas and holiday festivities. I danced at every opportunity. Michael, Marcus, Emile and Angelique all shared in the joyful spirit. We were harmoniously united again, eagerly anticipating 'our' baby's arrival in January.

Everyone had an input in naming the baby. After much lighthearted and serious debate, we finally agreed to call her Athena Christiana Aclima—names that satisfied everyone. My mother and aunt also decided to come to Florida for the birth to assist wherever and whenever necessary. This was an exciting time. Notwithstanding all this action, I kept my focus on my preparation. My daily routine was set and I made sure that I followed my checklist, especially my hypno-meditation practice.

At this point, my fears had all diminished and I no longer felt anxiety about any possible aspect of the birthing process. In my head and in my heart, I had turned my negatives into positives – even the possibility of a caesarean section or death.

I applied myself diligently to living by the motto "Do your best and let God do the rest". I focused wholeheartedly on strengthening my connection with God so that I could feel His guidance and presence every step of the way. I imagined that Mary must have strongly felt this way during her birthing of Jesus.

Then the 'big day' arrived. My amniotic membrane broke at 5 a.m. Mike excitedly announced to all, "The show is on the road. Wake up! Wake up!" Emile rushed into the bedroom with the borrowed stethoscope to begin checking the baby's heartbeat which he kept monitoring while I relaxed and allowed the mild contractions to flow. Michael, Marcus, and Emile timed my contractions. Angelique checked to make sure that everything was in my bags for the hospital and that her room was prepared for the new baby. My mother and aunt fixed breakfast for me and the family. Everyone was involved in this performance and I was the star. What a wonderful feeling! I was determined and confident that I would give my best performance and would not disappoint anyone. Besides, God was leading my team.

We followed the set procedures and contacted the doctors. I rested comfortably at home until the contractions were stronger and 5 minutes apart. Then, at 9:30 a.m. we went to the hospital and complied with their routine. Mike remained in the labor room with me while the others waited in the waiting room. Throughout the labor, I focused on my breathing, went into a deeper level of consciousness, and communicated loving, reassuring messages to my baby. I visualized my baby properly positioned to birth normally and I felt the loving presence of God within me.

I welcomed each contraction as a surge of Divine energy flowing through me and visualized my pelvic muscles gently moving to accommodate the passage of my baby. I felt totally comfortable with how my labor was progressing.

Then a nurse insensitively shook me out of my peaceful state to get me to sign an agreement for an epidural. Mike protested strongly while I asserted that I was not signing that agreement because I did not want an epidural and that I had already informed them about my decision.

At this point, there was another contraction which felt very painful and I had to struggle to flow with it since I was feeling annoyed and distracted by the nurse who had disturbed me. After that, I quickly returned to my peaceful, meditative state and the labor continued to progress smoothly, so smoothly that Michael fell asleep in the chair next to me.

The doctor came in at around 11:00 a.m. and was disappointed that I was not ready to deliver. She expected that I would deliver before lunch time. So she decided to speed up my contractions by putting me on the Pitocin drip. I did not resist even though I would have preferred not to have it.

Instead, I concentrated more on God's presence, my baby and flowing with the contractions which were getting stronger. An internal monitor was placed within me. At that point I told the doctor that I would not be having this baby before lunch so that she would leave me alone. She didn't need any convincing about that since she seemed in a hurry to leave anyway. Mike then left to give the rest of the family this information and to suggest that they also go home for lunch. He must have spent a few minutes with them.

I was alone in the labor room, quietly giving full attention to this stage of the birthing. I became an observer while being fully conscious of what was taking place within me. There was an intense pressure and movement in my pelvic area. I realized that my baby was 'bearing down'.

Just then, the nurse arrived and realized what was happening. She moved into action and was hurriedly transporting me to the delivery room when I glimpsed Michael slowly walking down the corridor. He broke into a trot when he saw me and was given a gown to wear as he accompanied me into the delivery room.

My focus was now totally on my baby and on controlling my pushing so that it would be an easy delivery for my baby and me. At this point all of my training kicked in. I kept mentally talking my baby through this passage and asking God to help me do it right. I was totally engrossed in my task at hand. My whole being was making a concerted effort and I can honestly say that I felt no pain, just an extreme tightness and a powerful urge to push. I heard the nurse telling me that the doctor would be coming soon and could I wait. I responded firmly, "No, you just deliver my baby now."

And she was delivered and arrived safely. I remember seeing first the expression on Mike's face. He was glowing with awe and delight (it was the first time that he had witnessed a birthing). Then I saw and held my baby. Words cannot describe the depth of joy, relief, and gratitude I felt.

That was truly a moment of pure ecstasy, my Olympic win! "Thank you, God! Thank you, God!" kept resounding in my mind. "My cup runneth over. Yes, God, we did it!"

Not even the doctor's indifferent attitude could affect my happiness. When the doctor eventually arrived, she began by reprimanding me for not waiting for her. I replied sweetly, "I waited nine months for this moment."

Then after a cursory examination, she questioned the nurse "She did not have an episiotomy?" To which Michael promptly responded, "And do you plan to give her one now?"

There were no lacerations. All was intact. The delivery was excellent from all reports. My baby was in good health except for some mild jaundice. Nothing to worry about. I felt on top of the world. No pain, no regrets – only positive memories of a very beautiful, magical, orgasmic experience.

Thank you, God, for helping me to be what you want me to be – A BIRTHING GODDESS.

We got it right!

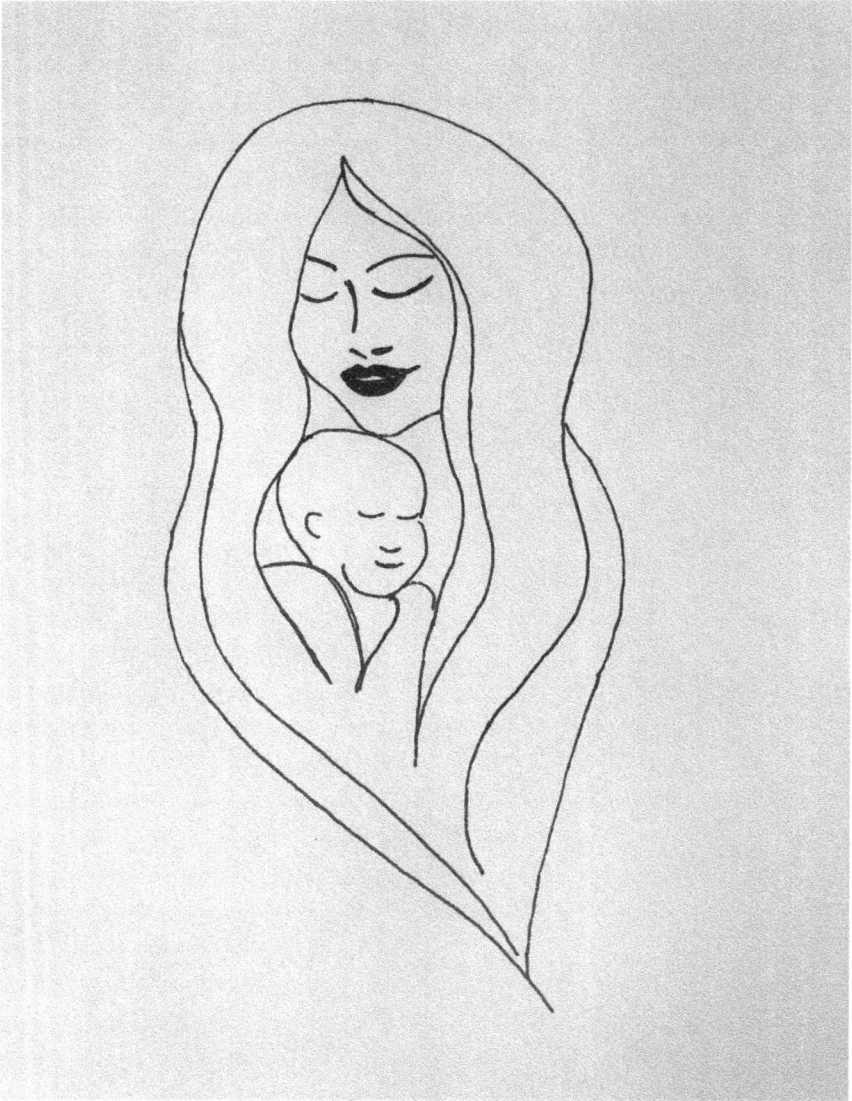

Chapter 2
Debriefing Myths

"Myths which are believed in tend to become true."
George Orwell (English novelist)

Pregnancy and birthing are not isolated events in our lives. They are influenced by many factors: beliefs, attitudes, experiences, health, spirituality, and cultural traditions to name a few. These factors can be based on myths or truths. Once they are embedded in the conscious and subconscious minds, they all become what I like to call *personal truths* which influence our thinking, our feelings, and our behavior during pregnancy and birthing.

If your personal truth is that pregnancy is a beautiful, exciting, and fulfilling period in a woman's life and that childbirth is an uplifting, spiritual experience, then you will wholeheartedly welcome and prepare for this event without any fears or resistance. In addition, when this personal truth is validated by scientific fact and empirical evidence, your reality will more than likely be a happy pregnancy and a normal, natural, comfortable, and joyful birthing experience.

If, on the other hand, your personal truth is that pregnancy is a difficult time in a woman's life and that natural birthing is a painfully horrific ordeal, then you will be filled with fears and resistance allowing this negative personal truth to inevitably become your reality. Unfortunately, this has been the experience of millions and millions of women who accept this negative belief as their personal truth. To make matters worse, this damaging personal truth is based on myths and propaganda. What a tragedy for women! We owe it to ourselves and to humanity to debrief ourselves of these noxious myths and propaganda that disempower us and rob us of the joys of our true birthright.

Let us look closely at the source of the most destructive myth that birthing is destined to be a very painful ordeal. History has shown that many interpreters of the Bible believe that this is the heritage of women as punishment for the original sin of Eve. Dr. Grantly Dick-Read, the renowned obstetrician, is one of many writers who challenge the biblical 'curse of Eve'. In his book, *childbirth without fear,* he produces compelling proof of inaccurate translations of words that create the scenario of painful childbirth. He cites research that has shown that the Hebrew words 'etzev' and 'itstsabon', initially used to describe childbirth, meant 'toil' and 'hard work'. But, in the Authorized Version of the Bible, these words were translated as 'pain'. This effectively put the stamp on childbirth as a painful tribulation that women must endure. The truth is that childbirth, like any other worthwhile task, does involve much toil, effort, and hard work. The woman who does not prepare herself physically, mentally, emotionally, and spiritually will more than likely experience pain during childbirth. But the woman who makes the effort to develop herself fully will be adequately prepared to cope comfortably with the hard work of birthing.

Those who study the Bible will note that nowhere in the Bible is there any documentation that Mary experienced pain while birthing Jesus. It appears that her body, mind, and spirit were well prepared for birthing. She harbored no fears and she enjoyed a normal, natural and safe delivery without medical intervention. She is our role model as the original Birthing Goddess.

A woman's total physiology was designed by our Divine Creator for birthing, which is a natural, normal function for a Birthing Goddess. As any medical practitioner will confirm, natural functions of a healthy body are not painful. Yet many women do experience painful natural birthing. What then are the main causes of this pain? **Inadequate preparation** of our total being for the hard work of birthing and the foreign element of **fearfulness** that is based mainly on the anticipation of a painful birthing experience.

Dr. Grantly Dick-Read, in his book *childbirth without fear*, has identified the fear-tension-pain syndrome and explains in detail how it works. To summarize: the emotion of fear triggers chemicals such as adrenaline which create tension in the body and especially in the birthing muscles. Tension prevents the muscles from relaxing and stretching to allow the birth channel to open and the muscles to work harmoniously to move the baby down and out. It is the tension from the excessive pressure on the birthing muscles and often the resulting tearing of the muscles that cause the pain. When there is no fear, natural birthing chemicals such as oxytocin are released to speed up the labor and allow the birthing muscles to relax and work as nature intended them to do. The chart in chapter 4 indicates clearly the significant differences between the process of a fearful birthing and a fear-free birthing.

It is easy to get sucked into this fear of birthing pain by the powerful negative programming that exists. We only need to listen to the graphic, horrendous stories of women's painful birthing experiences. We can hear the screams, see the twisted agonized faces of birthing women on T.V. shows and in movies, and feel great empathy and compassion for them. Yes, it is true that many women have experienced great pain during birthing. I, too, experienced pain while birthing my first three children because I had accepted this myth that pain is an inevitable and dreadful part of the normal birthing process. This was my personal truth at that time. I anticipated the pain and activated the powerful Law of Attraction. My belief became my reality. I experienced the pain that I attracted to myself.

Mythical beliefs are also reinforced by many medical practitioners, childbirth professionals, and hospitals that promote pregnancy as a medical condition and birthing as an affliction that needs pain-relieving interventions. But birthing is not meant to be a painful affliction.

Pregnancy and birthing are not normally medical conditions. They are healthy, natural processes in a woman. Health care-givers and medical practitioners serve simply to monitor the process and to identify and treat any medical condition that may develop during this time.

Hospitals and medical practitioners do little to help the mother-to-be to remove her fears and prepare herself properly for a natural pain-free birthing. Instead, they find it easier to readily offer several medical pain-relieving options. Both the epidural and cesarean deliveries are such options that involve the administering of an anesthetic.

The epidural is often routinely used even though there are several potential disadvantages and negative side effects to both mother and baby. An epidural usually causes a delay of the birth which can lead to other complications and possible medical interventions. In addition an epidural can deaden the pain as well as other sensations so that the mother is unable to have full control of her muscles to assist in the final stages of the birth. The baby's functioning is also affected, since whatever enters the mother's bloodstream also enters into the baby's circulation. For instance, it is well known that anesthesia can affect the baby's ability to suck right after birth.

The cesarean section offers freedom from birthing pain (the pain comes after the birth) and a quick, easy, convenient and secure delivery option. When you are due, you can simply schedule a cesarean section at a specific time and place convenient to you and the doctor. No need to wait for the natural process to begin. There are those who also feel that birthing by C-Section protects the vagina and keeps it intact for sexual activities. This is the lure of the C-section!

In our modern, fast-paced, civilized world, many women find it difficult to commit to the time and effort needed to prepare themselves fully for pain-free, natural birthing. It is no surprise then that cesarean deliveries are growing at an outrageous rate. I often wonder if women are being seriously misled into believing that a C-Section is better or safer than a normal, vaginal birth. Is this why many women are agreeing so easily to having a C-Section and settling for an elective cesarean?

The truth is that a well-prepared, healthy woman is fully empowered to birth her baby without pain, medical intervention, or damage to her vaginal muscles which can be returned to improved functioning with regular Kegel exercises.

The fact is that a C-Section is major abdominal surgery and involves far greater short and long term risks to mother and baby than vaginal births. Up-to-date information on all the risks and hazards of a C-Section is readily available in books and on the internet. Become very knowledgeable about this option before you make your choice. This medical intervention totally disempowers a woman during birthing. A woman relinquishes her God-given power to the medical practitioners when her baby is delivered by a C-Section. By adopting a passive role during birthing a woman loses much of the fulfillment and joy of participating fully in the actual birth of her baby since both mother and baby are medicated with the anesthetic. This also makes it harder for mother and baby to bond and for the onset of breastfeeding. In addition, because of the surgery, there is inevitably a longer recovery time.

A C-Section becomes necessary only in exceptional cases when there are health problems and the life of the parent or child is at risk.

The biggest myth of all is that women cannot achieve the power of a Birthing Goddess and enjoy birthing her baby naturally without pain. It is this seed of doubt that is implanted by others that prevents us from persevering towards the goal of a pain-free birth. It robs us of the 100% commitment needed to develop our total being. It takes a tremendous, consistent effort to debrief our minds of the negative programming that has permeated our subconscious being. We can truly understand the powerful effect of all that we have experienced from the moment of our conception and throughout our childhood. We are the product of all our experiences. We absorb without question all that is fed to us—until we become empowered to challenge the negative programming and choose more authentic, positive beliefs.

As adults we do have that power. We have the ability to learn, to gain knowledge, to change and to develop all our capacities in a balanced manner, and to make informed, wiser choices for ourselves and for the benefit of others. We can recognize why we think the way we think, why we feel the way we feel, why we behave the way we behave and why we are the way we are. That is the essential first step.

Then we can choose to change. We can do that without regret or allocation of blame for our present state of functioning. Regrets, guilt or blame are all negative forces which can hold us back. There are many ways in which we can cancel, transform, or at least minimize these negative feelings so that we can clear the path towards a more positive goal ahead of us.

In the following chapters you will find effective techniques to help you to do just that.

It is your 100% commitment that is needed now.

You must believe in your God-given ability. Trust in the Higher Power within you to manage and cancel the man-made limitations set on your aspirations. Strengthen your inner motivation by reading inspirational books such as Louise Hay's *The Power Is within You*, Marianne Williamson's *A Woman's Worth*, and Dr. Wayne Dyer's *You'll See It When You Believe It* or listening to inspirational audio tapes.

Personal empowerment is such a wonderful feeling. We owe it to ourselves to use every opportunity to develop our capabilities and reclaim our birthright as Birthing Goddesses. The information and exercises in this book can help you to achieve this honorable goal.

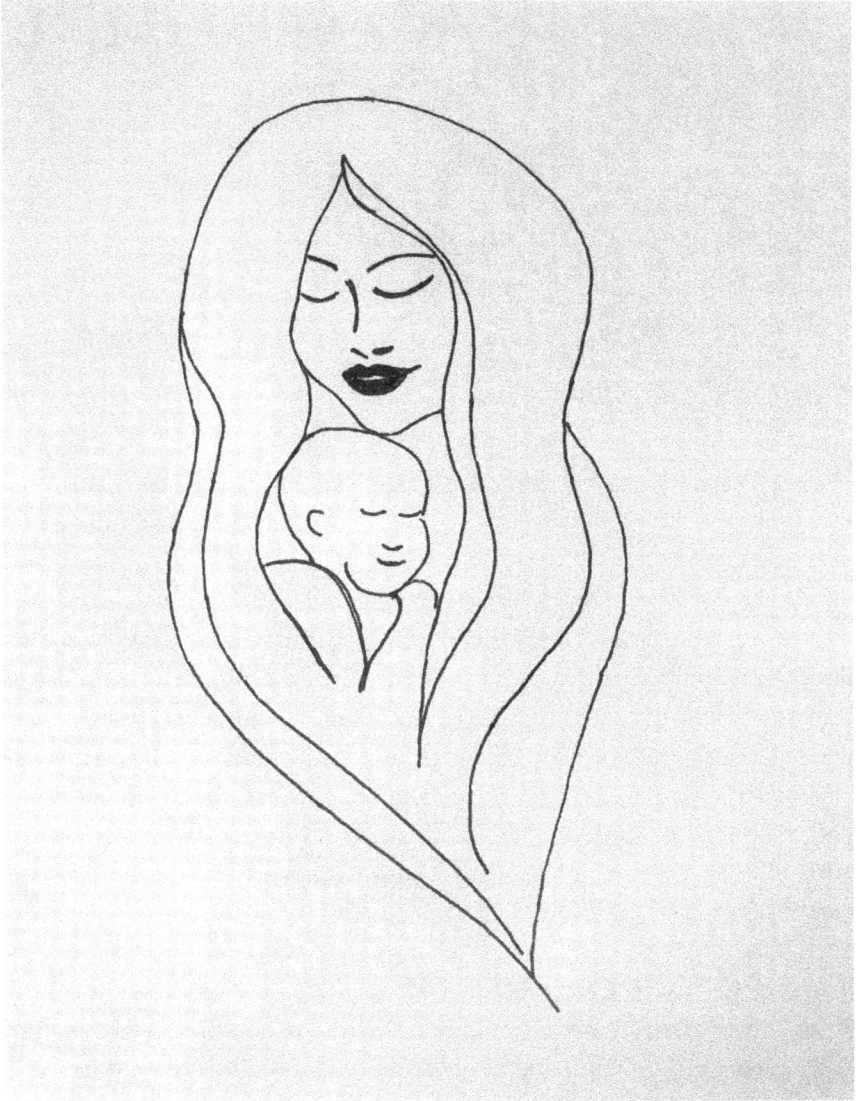

Chapter 3
Honoring Your Body

"The body is shaped, disciplined, honored and in time trusted".
Martha Graham

Preparing your body for pregnancy and childbirth means honoring your body, probably more than you have ever done. It is your body that will be nuturing the growth of your child. Bringing a child into the world is a strenuous affair and demands physical fitness. Your general health and body must be kept in good condition and your birthing muscles must be trained to be flexible and well toned. In addition, you will need to develop the ability to control your breathing and all your muscles so that you can relax and ultimately trust your body to facilitate the birthing process.

THE POWER OF BREATH

With breath there is life in your body, without breath there is no life. A simple fact. And yet many people take breathing for granted, since it is an automatic biological function. This is probably why so many of us have allowed ourselves to develop poor breathing habits without realizing the effect on our health. Studies have found that there is a direct link between our breathing patterns and our level of health. Bad breathing patterns such as shallow chest breathing, mouth breathing, and over-breathing are responsible for most respiratory ailments such as asthma, sleep apnea, and sinusitis.

Good breathing patterns such as diaphragmatic breathing, circular breathing and patterned breathing are all forms of conscious breathing and when done properly promote a healthy body, mind and spirit.

A mother-to-be who consciously develops strong healthy breathing patterns will have better fitness during her pregnancy and for childbirth. In his book, *Magical Beginnings, Enchanted Lives*, Deepak Chopra states "Breathing is the bridge between your mind, body, and baby."

By making a conscious effort to practice healthy breathing, you will provide high quality oxygen that is essential for your baby's developing cells. In addition, you will be furnishing your baby with vital life force energy from the air you breathe. Remember that the breath of life is the spiritual connection with our Divine Creator providing us with both oxygen and life energy.

There are numerous healthy breath techniques, but we will be focusing on the ones that are most effective for you during pregnancy and birthing.

Deep Abdominal Breathing

This is the fundamental healthy breathing pattern, and most other beneficial breathing techniques are variations of this. Abdominal breathing is a return to the powerful deep breathing we were born with. Just look at the way a sleeping baby breathes. Notice how his abdomen rises as he breathes in (like a balloon filling with air) and how his abdomen falls as he breathes out. This is also called natural breathing or diaphragmatic breathing.

Most adults have forgotten how to breathe deeply and instead use shallow breaths into the upper part of the chest rather than the abdomen. During labor, shallow chest breathing limits the oxygen supply to bodily tissues and this tends to induce pain. Shallow breathing also increases anxiety which in turn, increases the pain. Chest breathing is usually at a fast pace. This rapid expansion and contraction of the chest cavity actually causes oxygen to bind too tightly to the hemoglobin molecules, constricting blood vessels and resulting in a decrease of oxygen and energy released to the body. The effect on the laboring mother is extreme exhaustion.

The good news is that everyone can easily and consciously return to a healthier deep abdominal breathing.

General benefits of deep abdominal breathing:
Deep abdominal breathing increases the quantity and quality of oxygen that goes into your blood stream to fully oxygenate your body and that of your baby. Chest breathing brings on the average a pint of fresh air to the lungs. Deep breathing increases this amount dramatically to between three or four pints and accomplishes the following:

- Activates the lymphatic system that removes and destroys dead cells and toxic material from your body, thereby cleansing your system.
- Allows your body to fully exchange incoming oxygen with out-going carbon dioxide.
- Increases the life force (psychic energy) and power that energizes both mother and baby.
- Acts upon the parasympathetic system which has a calming influence on the nervous system.
- Releases tension in the muscles and helps the body to relax.
- Acts continuously upon the diaphragm which then effects a gentle massage on the liver, stomach, spleen, and part of the intestines.
- Becomes a life skill to effectively reduce the stresses in everyday situations.
- Decreases the likelihood of post-natal depression.

Specific benefits of deep abdominal breathing during birthing:

- The steady rhythm of deep breathing is very calming during labor.
- Deep breathing becomes an automatic response to the surges.
- Contractions become more effective as birthing muscles are relaxed and move into place easily.
- Deep breathing provides you with a measure of self control, focus, and well-being.

- It allows you to rest and relax between contractions while providing you and your baby with additional vital supplies of oxygen and energy.

The Technique for Slow Abdominal Deep Breathing:

1. Begin by making yourself comfortable, lying on your back or sitting.
2. Place your hands over your stomach with your fingers barely touching. Good breathers start by *exhaling* with their stomachs compressed.
3. Exhale through your nostrils so that your lungs are almost empty and your stomach contracts. Your fingertips will touch.
4. Now breathe in slowly and deeply, consciously pushing the air to fill up your stomach so it expands and your fingertips separate.
5. Exhale slowly until your stomach contracts and your fingertips touch.
6. Continue consciously breathing this way, in and out through your nostrils slowly and deeply. Notice your stomach slowly expanding with the in-breath and contracting with the out-breath.
7. Breathe in to the count of four and out to the count of four. Allow your breathing to become slow, smooth, and rhythmical.

Practice. Practice. Practice! You can practice lying, sitting, standing, or walking so that this breathing pattern becomes natural to you. The benefits to your total health will be well worth the effort that you put into it. The more natural that this deep breathing becomes for you the easier it will be to employ it during labor as a relaxation and pain reducing technique.

Mastering this breathing method will benefit you, not only during pregnancy and labor, but also for the rest of your life. It is an essential life skill that gives you the energy you need to perform at your best. All professional athletes understand the importance of this and make it a fundamental part of their training. You too can make it a fundamental part of your birthing training.

Using deep breathing for relaxation: The 2:1 ratio

After you have gained control of the diaphragmatic movement, you can easily refine this technique by using a 2:1 ratio.

Exhale to the count of 4 and inhale to the count of 2. To relax even more deeply, exhale to the count of 8 and inhale to the count of 4.

During labor this is the deep breathing technique that will be very effective between your surges when you need to rest, relax, and provide your body and baby with an increased supply of oxygen and energy. At this time you can also close your eyes and focus on visualizing your inner sanctuary or a peaceful scene. This enhances your rest and relaxation time. It will also release any residual mental, emotional and physical tension after the surge is over, and it signals to you and your partner that the surge is beginning or ending.

This is also the technique you will use to center yourself before self-hypnosis or a meditation session.

Surge Breathing:

Surge Breathing is another variation of abdominal breathing. It involves slower, more focused breathing that coincides with the movement and pace of each surge. You will breathe in at a very slow, steady, and smooth pace, expanding your abdomen, in harmony with the surge. Try not to hold your breath. Keep it flowing smoothly. Take another breath if necessary. The important thing here is to breathe into your surge and keep your focus on filling up your abdomen with air. As the surge recedes, very slowly exhale. Focus on gently breathing down oxygen and energy to your uterus, and your baby, to facilitate the birthing process.

Surge breathing assists all your birthing muscles to work more efficiently, and shortens the length of labor. This technique needs regular and conscientious practice since it involves discipline and focus. Practice daily before you go to bed or first thing in the morning, increasing the length of your inhalation and exhalation while imagining you are fully expanding your abdomen in harmony with your surges. You will also get several opportunities to practice in your third trimester when you experience Braxton Hicks surges (often called 'practice contractions') that are irregular and painless.

Expulsion Breathing:

When you feel the urge to push, you will find that you will be focusing more on longer exhalations and shorter inhalations. Remember to put the tip of your tongue at the place where your front teeth and palate meet. This helps the pelvic floor to relax. Imagine your cervix opening as petals of a flower. Focus on your perineum relaxing and stretching to accommodate your baby. As you breathe out you will be using the power of your mind to send your thoughts, your breath, your energy and your love to your baby and all your birthing muscles so that your baby moves gently down and out into your arms.

This is another breathing variation that you will want to practice daily as you get to the end of your third trimester. By this time you will be gaining good control of your breath.

Quantum Touch Breathing:

This is based on the principle that energy follows thought. As I said earlier the breath provides us with oxygen as well as energy. The Chinese call this vital energy *Chi*; the Japanese call it *Ki*, the Yogis call it *Prana,* the Polynesians call it *Mana,* and in Hebrew it is called *Ruach.*

As you breathe you can use your mind to control the direction and strength of energy flowing into your body and out your body. This energy can then be directed wherever it is needed for healing and relieving pain. This is called '*running energy*'. Quantum Touch is one of the therapies that teach you to do this. You can learn more about this amazingly simple and effective technique by reading the book, *Quantum-Touch, The Power to Heal* by Richard Gordon. Better yet, try to attend a week-end training session.

I attended a Quantum Touch training program where I learned this easy and valuable technique. So, of course I used it on anyone who needed relief from headaches, pains, and discomfort with surprisingly successful results. I not only used it to help relieve discomfort in my pregnant daughter-in-law, but I also taught it to her during our hypno-meditation practice sessions so that she could then use it to relieve her own physical discomforts. Here we have another technique that can help to ease and eliminate pain during pregnancy and birthing with no detrimental side effects. More power to you!

Alternate Breathing:

Here is another breathing technique that you will find very useful during your pregnancy if you are experiencing nervous tension, anxiety, stress, or when you feel scattered or mentally blocked.

Benefits of Alternate Breathing:

- It acts like a sedative on the nervous system (without any negative side effects).
- It forces you to breathe slowly, and this in itself has a calming effect.
- It increases the capacity of the lungs.
- It balances the hemispheric functioning of the brain so you can utilize *whole brain thinking*.
- It improves your concentration and focus and your ability to think creatively.

Alternate breathing technique:

1. Sit comfortably with your spinal column straight and supple.
2. Rest the index and middle fingers of the right hand on the space between the two eyebrows. Press your ring finger against the left nostril, closing it and gently exhaling through the right nostril, counting to 6 (or about 6 seconds) mentally as you exhale. Then inhale immediately through the same nostril for a count of 6.
3. Now press the thumb gently against the right nostril, closing it off, and at the same time release the pressure on the left nostril. Exhale for a count of 6, and then inhale for a count of 6 through the left nostril.
4. Close the left nostril and open the right. Exhale and inhale for a count of 6 in the right nostril. Close the right and open the left nostril. Exhale and inhale to the count of 6 in the left nostril. Continue this round one more time so that you have done three rounds in total.

I find this exercise particularly helpful when I feel flustered. It is very easy to do, takes only a little time, and works quickly and effectively.

Yoga philosophy says, *"Mastering the breath brings mastery of life."* When you master your breathing you bring focus to the mind; energy and oxygen to the body cells; and strength and power to the muscles. Your performance and endurance will increase. This is the power source that enables trained martial arts practitioners to comfortably and painlessly smash through concrete bricks.

This is the power source that you can use more beneficially to bring forth your baby into this life with comfort and ease.

REST AND RELAXATION

'Releasing the Brakes'

There is a difference between rest and relaxation. You may lie in bed taking a rest or sit in a chair looking at TV and still be holding tension in your body and mind. You may be physically 'resting' but your mind and body may not necessarily be relaxed. Relaxation involves a conscious effort to release stress and tension in your mind and body.

Pregnancy is a time of additional stress and anxiety. Research done by the Fetal and Neo-Natal Stress Research Group (FNSRG) has clearly shown that stress and anxiety experienced by a pregnant woman is transmitted to her fetus. Increased stress hormones easily cross the placenta, flow through the umbilical cord, and can negatively affect the development of the fetus.

Now more than ever, it is important to learn to relax for your own well-being as well as the healthy development of your baby. An effective relaxation routine will not only help you to handle the stresses and anxieties of pregnancy but also to manage the level of tension in your body and mind during the actual birthing process.

Tensing your muscles during labor is like driving your car with your brakes on: The car slows down and is unable to go at full speed; more gas and effort is needed for the car to move forward, the engine strains and can be damaged. In the same way when you tense your birthing muscles, you slow down the process of labor. You then have to use much more energy and effort to birth your baby and run the risk of straining or tearing your muscles and inducing pain. In his book *childbirth without fear,* Dr. Grantly Dick-Read states *"The only pain stimulus that the uterus can record is excessive tension or actual tearing of tissues."*

Everyone can learn to relax the body and mind. There are many techniques to do so. I will describe here some of the ones that I find easy and most effective to use during pregnancy. Try them all and then choose and practice the ones that are best suited to you. You will note that all these relaxation techniques work with the conscious involvement of both the body and the mind.

Benefits that relaxation can bring to you:

- It reduces the level of tension and stress in your body and mind.
- It increases your energy level during pregnancy, birthing and after the birth.
- You will experience an improved quality of sleep, especially in the third trimester.
- You become more sensitive to your body and your baby.
- It increases your feeling of peace and security.
- It reduces the risk of high blood pressure during pregnancy.
- You experience less aches and pains due to muscle tension.
- It shortens labor.
- It helps you to rest and relax between contractions.
- It prevents tearing.
- It reduces the effects of fatigue during pregnancy, birthing and after the birth.
- It blocks the Fear-Tension – Pain cycle.

Guidelines for your relaxation routine:

- Choose a quiet place where you will not be disturbed.
- Try to practice at the same time each day—every morning or every evening. A regular pattern helps.

- Empty your bladder before you begin.
- Always make yourself comfortable before you begin. Choose a position that is best for you in your varying stages of pregnancy – lying on your back, semi-reclining, side-lying, or sitting.
- Use an audio-guided relaxation to assist you. You may find it easier to learn with an audio. Or you can have your partner guide you with the scripts that I offer.

Progressive Relaxation:

This relaxation technique was first developed by the American physiologist Dr. Edmund Jacobson. It is a good relaxation exercise to begin with since it helps to familiarize you with what your muscles feel like when they are tense and then how they feel when they are relaxed. You will be using all six muscle groups in your body. Step by step you will be consciously tensing and releasing one muscle group after another until you achieve total relaxation of your body.

At first, this exercise takes effort and concentration, but with regular practice you will be able to achieve total muscular relaxation easily and quickly without having to deliberately tense your muscles before you relax them.

Technique:

- Lie flat on your back on the floor, or any firm surface, with your arms at your side and your legs slightly apart. You may also choose a semi-reclining, side-lying, or sitting position.
- Close your eyes.
- Breathe slowly and deeply. Take deep, slow, abdominal breaths for a minute or two.
- Begin now:

Muscle Group 1 – Relaxing Your Arms

1. Close and clench the fist of your right hand.

2. Tighten your fist as much as you can. Feel the tension. Hold for a few seconds.

3. Release your fist and feel your fingers relax. Tighten your fist again and then tighten all the muscles in your right hand and arm. Hold for a few seconds.

4. Notice the tension.

5. Release and relax your arm and fist, allowing them to go totally limp. Feel the relaxation. Now do the same sequence with your left fist and arm.

Notice the difference in the sensations of tension and relaxation.

Muscle Group 2 – Relaxing Your Legs

1. Press your legs tightly against each other. Draw back your toes and push forward on your heels so that the muscles of your feet, calves and thighs are stretched and tensed.

2. Hold that pressure for a few seconds. Release and relax your legs so that they fall back limp into a position of rest.

3. Feel the relaxation. Do this several times if needed until you feel no tension in your legs.

Muscle Group 3 – Relaxing Your Abdomen, Buttocks and Pelvis

1. Breathe out slowly, sucking in your stomach as though you were trying to attach your stomach wall to your backbone.

2. Hold for a few seconds and feel the tension.

3. Release, relax and allow the air to refill your lungs naturally. Feel the relaxation in your stomach.

4. Squeeze your buttocks tightly until it lifts slightly off the floor. Hold, release, and relax.

5. Tighten the muscles of your pelvic floor. Hold. Release and note the feeling of relaxation as your muscles go loose and limp.

Muscle Group 4 – Relaxing Your Chest

1. Breathe in deeply and expand your chest. Hold.
2. Feel the tension and tightness in your chest.
3. Breathe out slowly through your nostrils, allowing your chest to relax and flatten and notice the relaxation in your chest.

Muscle Group 5 – Relaxing Your Back and Shoulders

1. Arch your back slightly and push back to bring your shoulder blades together. Hold.
2. Release and let your shoulders relax and go limp.
   Note the difference between the tension and the relaxation.

Muscle Group 6 – Relaxing Your Head and Neck

1 Tighten the muscles of your neck as if you were trying to lengthen your neck. Feel the tension and hold. Release and relax.

2 Clench your teeth and tighten the muscles of your jaw. Hold. Release and relax.

3 Squeeze your eyes tightly. Hold. Release and keep them gently closed. Feel your eyelids limp.

4 Tighten your forehead and scalp muscles. Hold. Release and enjoy the relaxed feeling in your whole head, face, neck and body.

Now focus on your deep diaphragmatic breathing, simply following the breath in and following the breath out. Allow your mind to travel over your body in each of the muscle groups, removing all small remaining tensions. Take a few more minutes to enjoy this feeling of being totally relaxed.

When you are ready, take three deep breaths, open your eyes on the third breath, exhale and gently stretch.

Always take your time returning to activity after a relaxation routine.

By systematically relaxing your body from head to toe, you increase the ability of your mind to focus on every part of your body and will it to relax without first having to consciously tense each individual body part. With regular practice, your mind will be able to induce relaxation at the very first sign of tension in any muscle of your body. You will then have greater control of your muscles.

Breathing Relaxation:

Here we will be using the deep abdominal breathing with the 2:1 ratio that I described earlier in this chapter. We will integrate this breathing into the systematic relaxation of each muscle group – breathing out tension and breathing in oxygen and life-force (pranic) energy.

Technique:

1. Sit or lie in a comfortable position. Close your eyes gently.
2. Begin by exhaling as slowly as you can to the count of 8, allowing your stomach to contract.
3. Now inhale to the count of 4 and feel your stomach expanding as it fills up with air. Continue with this pattern of breathing until your breathing becomes smooth and rhythmical.
4. Focus on your arms and hands. As you exhale, feel the tension flowing out and away from your hands. Allow them to go limp. As you inhale feel the life energy and oxygen filling and nourishing your arms.
5. Now systematically focus on all your other muscle groups, exhaling out tension and inhaling life energy and oxygen. Pay extra attention to any area of your body that still feels tense.
6. Continue breathing in this way. As you inhale, allow your whole body to experience this refreshing breath flowing into your body like a gentle wave. As you exhale, visualise this slow soothing wave removing and washing away all tension from your entire body. Enjoy this feeling of relaxation and rejuvenation.
7. When you are ready you can open your eyes and stretch gently.

Practice this relaxation exercise regularly so that you can use it effectively between the surges during labor when you need to rest, re-energize, and re-oxygenate your body and that of your baby.

Relaxation with Breath, Imagery, and Sound:

Physical, mental and emotional relaxation is made more effective with the use of breath, peaceful imagery, and soft tranquil music.

Technique:

- Combine your breath work with any of the visualizations described in Chapter 4, "The Magic of Mental Power."
- Add your favorite affirmations.
- Play tranquil music in the background.

You will find that your relaxation will become more profound and even more beneficial to you and your baby.

Massage and Touch Relaxation:

Another effective way of relaxing your body and mind is through massages.

A Pregnancy massage by a trained masseur is therapeutic body-work. It enhances the function of muscles and joints, improves blood circulation and general body tone and relieves mental and physical stress. It is a form of soft tissue massage that can alleviate many of the common muscular aches and pains experienced during pregnancy.

The Light-Touch massage is particularly beneficial in the later stages of pregnancy and especially during birthing. It induces relaxation and helps to relieve discomfort. In addition it can normalize heart rate and blood pressure. This Light-Touch technique was developed by Constance Palinsky after much research into pain management. It was found that a light-touch massage, that may cause goose bumps to arise, stimulates the secretion of endorphins (the happy hormones) and oxytocin which facilitates nature's birthing process. The advantages of this light-touch massage are several: it is safe, non-invasive, and can easily be learned by anyone. Both you and your partner can use this technique and have fun doing it to each other.

The Light-Touch Technique:

The person receiving the massage should assume a comfortable position. For example, the expectant mother can sit on a birth ball or in a chair learning forward with her head resting on a pillow at the side of the bed; or she might prefer to lie on her side or on her back—whatever is most comfortable at that time.

The giver also gets into a comfortable position: Using only the fingertips, fingernails or the back of the fingers, gently and lightly stroke the skin on the arms, legs, neck, shoulders, or any other parts of the body. During the birthing, stroke the abdomen in a wide circular pattern between surges to encourage relaxation of abdominal muscles. When stroking the back, begin either at the base of the spine and stroke upward and outward to the side of the body in a V pattern, or begin at the nape of the neck and stroke downward in an inverted V formation, from the spine toward the sides. This is enjoyable and particularly relaxing for the birthing mother.

Acupressure and **Reflexology** are other touch techniques that can also release tension from the body and promote relaxation and a higher level of wellness. Explore these options and use the ones that are most effective for you. The important thing is to be aware of the stress and tension signals in your body and to alleviate them in the appropriate way before it becomes damaging to you and your developing baby.

Take charge of your own wellbeing. A relaxed and calm disposition will help you to enjoy your pregnancy more fully.

EXERCISE

Prenatal daily exercise is important for a healthy pregnancy.

Safe exercise can maintain and increase your fitness level during pregnancy and prepare you for a pain free easier childbirth.

General Benefits of Prenatal Exercise:

- It strengthens your muscles.
- It lessens the common discomforts of pregnancy such as back pain, swelling, fatigue, and constipation.
- It boosts your energy levels.
- It releases stress.
- It helps you to relax and sleep better.
- It tones and relaxes the birthing muscles.
- It prevents urinary incontinence.
- It shortens labor.
- It eliminates postpartum blues.
- It speeds up the return to pre-pregnancy weight.

A note of caution: Be careful that your exercise, as with any other activity that you engage in, is safe for you and your baby. Ensure that you have no health conditions that may bar you from certain physical activities. Avoid contact sports and those with an increased potential for falls such as horse back riding and gymnastics.

Regular exercisers can modify their routine and still maintain general fitness.

Safe Prenatal Exercises

Walking
Get some good walking shoes and walk as often as you can – early morning or late afternoon. This is also a good opportunity to practice your rhythmical abdominal breathing and introduce your baby to the beauty of nature. Walking strengthens your legs, tones your body and refreshes your total being.

Swimming
Swimming is one of the best pregnancy exercises as the water supports your weight and balance problems are greatly reduced. This is a great exercise for total fitness and can be done throughout your pregnancy.

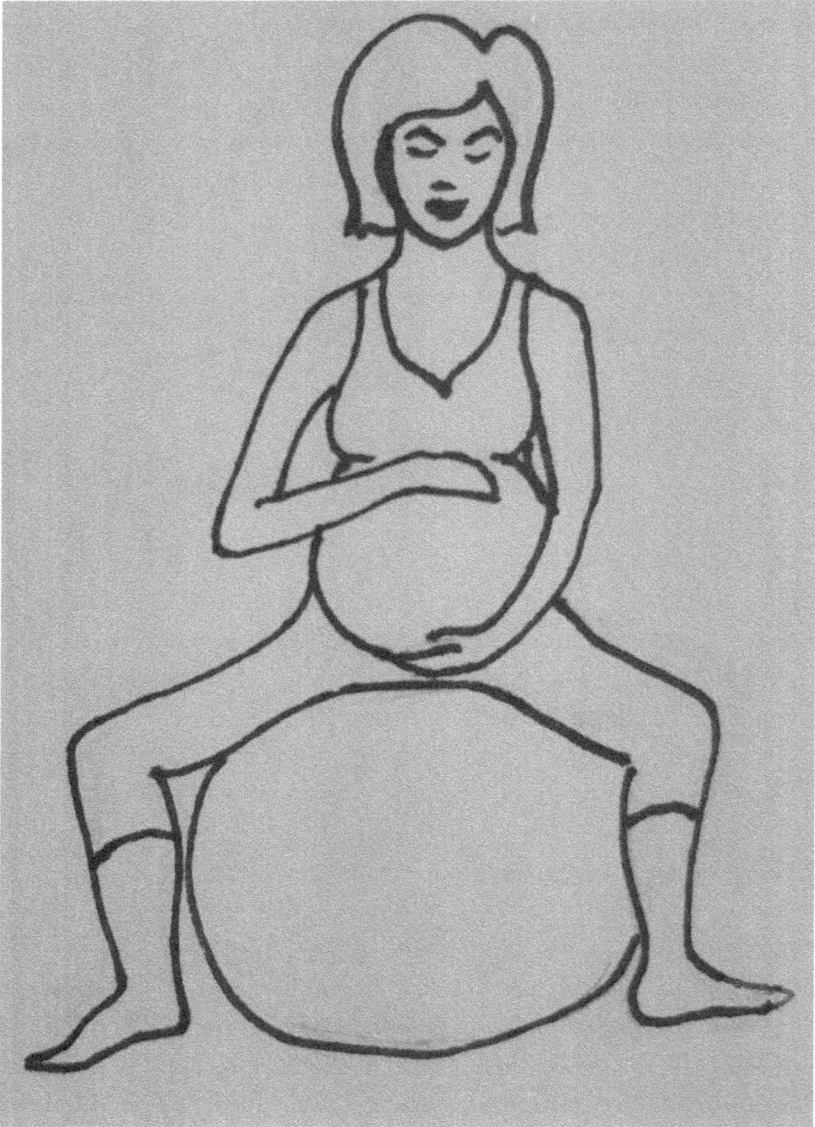

The Birthing Ball

The birth ball is a prenatal exercise tool that is fun to use. You will also find it helpful during labor. If you plan to use one, get a professional birth ball, not the toy balls for children.

Benefits of the Birthing Ball

- It tones and strengthens your inner thighs, legs, and pelvic region (critical birthing muscles).
- It strengthens lower back and abdominal muscles.
- It promotes good posture which gives extra room for your baby to maintain the preferred anterior position in the womb.
- In addition it is invaluable during labor:
  - o The rhythmic movement of the ball is great for relaxing both you and the baby as it releases tension in your back.
  - o It speeds up the birthing process as it encourages your baby to move down and out, taking advantage of gravity since you are in an upright position.

There are many ways in which you can use a birthing ball since it is flexible yet firm. You can sit on it, hug it, use it as a back rest, and/or bounce gently on it.

When you sit on the birthing ball, keep your feet flat on the floor and about 2 feet apart. Hold on to both sides of the ball and then slowly roll your hips from side to side or use any other movement that feels good to you. You can sit on the ball rather than on a chair when looking at TV and use it as often as you can. After a while, you will probably find it more comfortable than slouching in a chair, especially during labor.

Yoga

Prenatal Yoga is particularly advantageous at this time. It promotes profound relaxation of body and mind. In addition, several of the poses focus on stretching, strengthening, and toning the specific muscles that are involved in labor and childbirth. I used Yoga as part of my childbirth training and I found it to be very beneficial, especially since I was able to incorporate breathing, self-hypnosis, visualization, and meditation into my practice sessions.

There are many Yoga training classes. Seek out an experienced Hatha Yoga teacher who will be able to guide you into the yoga poses that are safe and beneficial during pregnancy.

Here are a few of them that you can practice at home:

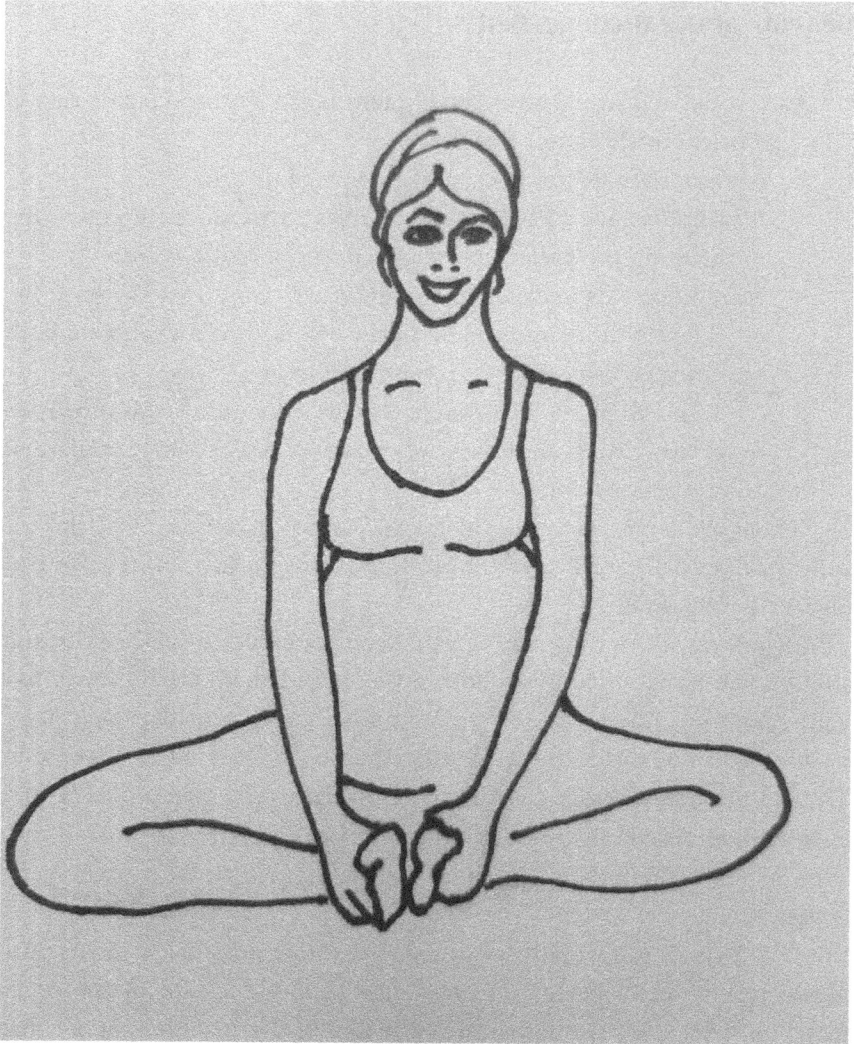

The Butterfly Position

Benefits:

This exercise stretches the muscles and ligaments in your pelvic girdle to make it more flexible in preparation for the passage of your baby. In addition it tones and strengthens your inner thighs.

Technique:

1. Sit on the floor or on a mat.
2. Bend your knees slightly and put the soles of your feet together.
3. Place your hands on your ankles and gradually draw your feet closer to your body.
4. Allow your elbows to rest on your knees and gently push your knees down so that you can feel your groin muscles stretching.
5. Hold your back straight.
6. Take a few slow, deep breaths and allow your tail bone to sink down to the ground and your thigh and leg muscles to stretch and relax.
7. Hold this position for 2 to 3 minutes.
8. Gently stretch your legs out and relax.

With regular practice you will be able to pull your heels close to your groin area and your knees will be able to drop closer to the ground, giving you the ultimate stretch and tone.

The Squatting Position

Benefits:

- It stretches and widens the pelvic opening.
- It stretches and lengthens the muscles around the hips and groin.
- It increases circulation in the pelvic area.
- It strengthens the inner thighs and legs.
- It relieves lower back pain.
- It can be used as a birthing position since it shortens the birth path and eases labor by making good use of gravity.

It reduces the chances for tearing of perineal tissues.

Technique:

- With feet slightly apart bend your knees and slowly squat down, keeping your feet and heels flat on the floor. (When first doing this, it may be difficult. I suggest you keep your back against a wall or have someone support you from behind.)
- Breathe slowly and deeply in this position, sending energy and oxygen to your pelvic muscles. You may hold this position for as long and as often as you can. Better yet – integrate it into your daily life: looking at TV, reading a book, or gardening. With practice it becomes a comfortable position.

During my pregnancy I used to squat with my back against a wall and do most of my studying this way. After a while, it became a preferred position.

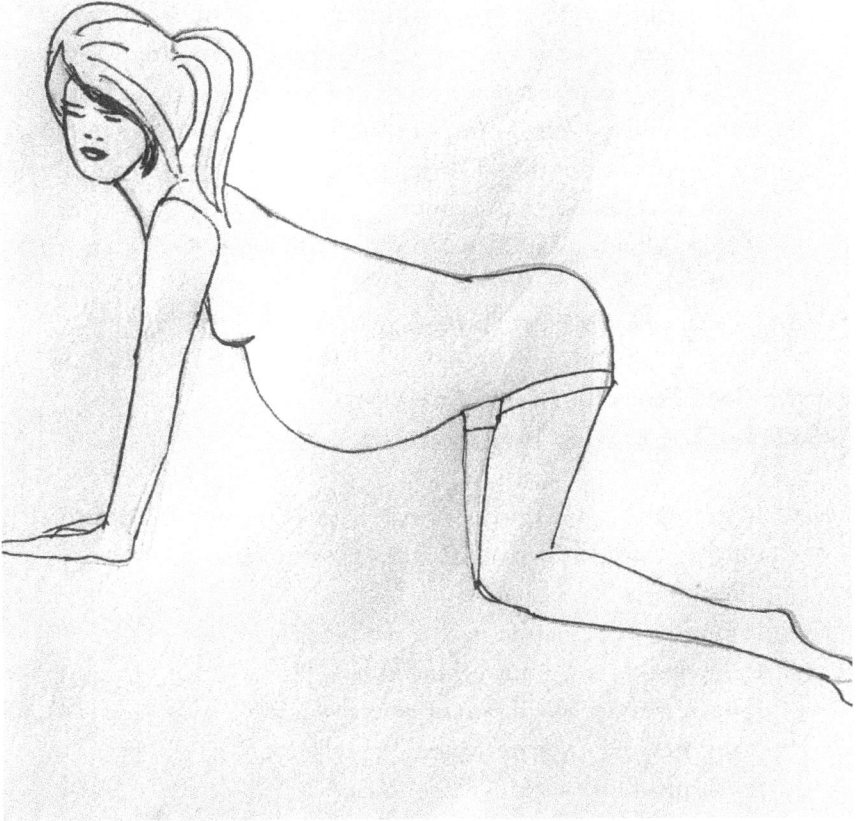

The Pose of the Cat
This exercise imitates the cat as it flexes and relaxes its spine

Benefits of the Pose of the Cat:

- It increases spinal flexibility.
- It corrects the pelvic tilt against gravity

It relieves back ache.

Technique:

1. Get into a hands and knees position with your hands directly under your shoulders and your knees directly under your hips.
2. Inhale deeply while raising your head and depressing your spine so that your back becomes concave. Hold for 2-3 seconds.
3. Exhale slowly while lowering your head and rounding your back into a convex position. Contract your abdomen and pull in your buttocks. Hold for 2-3 seconds.
4. Return slowly to the first position allowing your stomach to soften and fall.
5. Repeat this movement 5 times once or twice a day.

Pelvic Floor Exercise (Kegel Exercises)
Benefits of the Pelvic Floor Exercise:

- It strengthens and increases elasticity of pelvic muscles so that they will stretch easily with minimal trauma as your baby passes through the birth canal.
- It improves circulation in this area.
- It prevents urinary incontinence.
- It decreases the likelihood of hemorrhoids.
- It restores and improves vaginal muscle tone.
- It enhances love making.

Technique:

1. Empty your bladder before doing this exercise. This exercise may be done in any position.
2. Begin inhaling and tightening the muscles around your anus and vagina.
3. Pull the muscles up, squeezing steadily and pulling them up to your abdomen. Hold for 5-6 seconds.

4. Release slowly while exhaling.
   Do this at least 5 times.

Practice this exercise frequently everyday. Aim for 50 times a day. Just think of all the benefits of this simple and enjoyable exercise. Remember that the more you practice, the more beneficial it will be to you. Place some post-it notes throughout your home, work, and car to remind you to practice. You will be thrilled with the results!

Perineal Massage

This is another "must do" exercise to prevent tearing and pain.

Gently massage your perineal muscles with warm oil every day. Make it a part of your bath routine before you moisturize the rest of your body. Begin doing this at least two months before you are due. This will help your perineal rim and tissues to soften, relax, and stretch more easily over your baby's head during birth.

NUTRITION

Everything you eat or drink goes into your baby and will affect his/her development. **Your baby's healthy development depends on your health,** so you really have to be very mindful about what you eat and drink.

The main rule to remember is to keep your diet balanced and nutritious. That means eating a variety of foods and not too much of any one thing. Anything taken to the extreme becomes a negative. It also means cutting out or cutting down on junk foods, sodas, and snacks such as chips that are lacking in nutrition or have high fat, sugar or salt content.

There are many healthy substitutes on the market for you to choose from.

Here is a list of nutritious foods that you can have:

- Lots of fruits and vegetables
- Whole grain bread and cereals
- Lean meat, chicken and safe fish

- Dried peas, beans, nuts and seeds
- Low fat milk, cheese and yogurt
- Green leafy vegetables and salads
- Very small amounts of food high in fat, sugar, and salt content

During pregnancy, your body needs an increased supply of calcium, protein, iron, folic acid and vitamins. A balanced, healthy diet can meet your needs. But if you wish to use a prenatal dietary supplement, ensure that it does not have any undesired or harmful side effects.

Here is a list of foods that you should avoid:

- Junk foods
- Alcohol and caffeine
- Fatty and greasy foods
- Additives such as monosodium glutamate and saccharin
- Sushi
- Fish with elevated levels of methyl mercury, swordfish, shark, king mackerel
- Uncooked or cured meats
- Fad diets
- Drinks with artificial sweeteners

Morning sickness (nausea and vomiting) is a common experience during early pregnancy. Here are some tips that help to alleviate it:

- Eat some dry bread, crackers or cereal before getting up out of bed.
- Get up slowly without sudden movements.
- Avoid greasy and highly spiced foods.
- Try using ginger or the traveling sickness wrist band.

Weight Management

The American College of Obstetricians and Gynecologists recommend a weight increase of 3-4 lbs in the first 3 months, and then 3-4 lbs per month for the rest of the pregnancy. That is a weight gain of approximately 25–30 lbs.

The National Academy of Science recommends that you increase your daily caloric intake by 150 calories in the first trimester and 350 additional calories daily in the second and third trimester. It is true that you are eating for two, but that does not mean that you have to eat twice as much as you normally eat.

Eat and enjoy at least three balanced meals a day and smaller nutritious snacks throughout the day.

Water and Liquids

Water performs several important functions in your body such as transporting essential nutrients throughout your body, eliminating toxins and waste products, aiding digestion, maintaining a healthy body temperature and helping to prevent muscle cramps and constipation.

In between your meals drink lots and lots of plain, clean spring or filtered room – temperature water. Keep yourself and your baby well hydrated. Drink at least 10 glasses of water per day. In addition drink juice, milk, soy milk, or other nutritious drinks. Cheers!

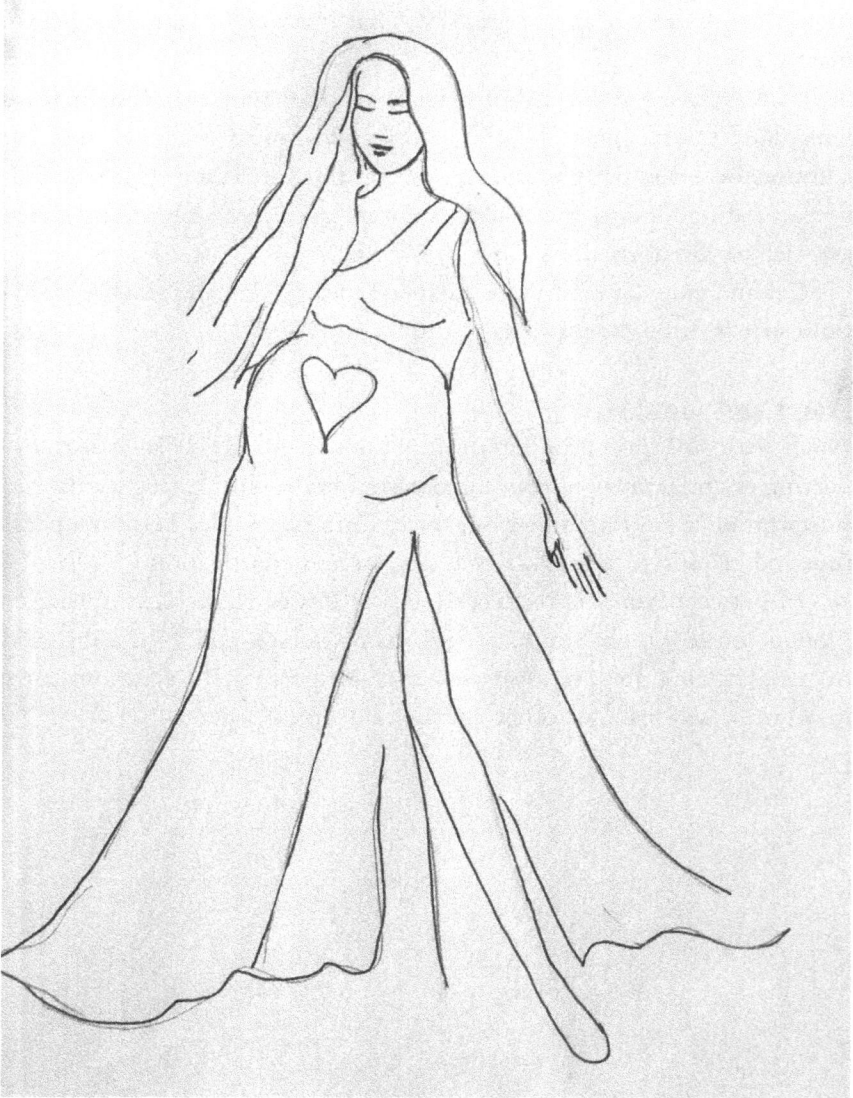

<u>**BODY CARE**</u>

Nourish and pamper your body. Treat it with sensitivity and love. You will be aware of many structural, biological, and physiological changes in your body – including the most obvious–your body shape.

Lovingly caress and moisturize your skin daily to maintain its elasticity. Get a weekly massage with your favorite aromatherapy oils. Your husband or partner can give you a light touch massage. Or a professional can give you a light or deep tissue, therapeutic prenatal massage. Your skin will glow, your body will feel relaxed, and you will feel wonderfully tranquil. A massage is good for your body, mind and spirit.

Do not forget your face. Give yourself a facial at least twice a month and keep looking radiant, beautiful and blooming. Smile often with gratitude and peace as you allow all the muscles in your face to relax. Your hair texture may even change so get a new easy to manage, and flattering hair style.

Dress in fashion with comfortable, attractive clothes. Do not hesitate to show off your new shape. No camouflage needed! You are a Birthing Goddess! Dress with pride and confidence.

Body care also involves monitoring the development of your baby and your own biological changes. So ensure that you get regular check-ups by your doctor, midwife or health care provider.

Feel free to explore complementary and alternative health care and therapies. Many of these therapies have not been subjected to stringent scientific studies, but empirical evidence certainly suggests that they offer effective help and do not have the damaging side effects of most medical interventions. For me, medical intervention is a last resort when other more natural means are not working.

Following is a list of some of these alternative and complementary health care therapies:

- Acupuncture
- Naturopathy
- Homeopathy
- Acupressure
- Reflexology
- Cranio-sacral Therapy
- Quantum Touch Healing

- Reiki
- Chiropractic Care

A special word about Chiropractic Care:

During pregnancy, vertebral misalignments can take place in your body due to a combination of hormonal changes that foster relaxation of ligaments and biomechanical changes. Chiropractic care throughout your pregnancy restores balance and alignment to your pelvic muscles and ligaments to relieve the stress, discomfort and pain misalignment causes. Spinal adjustment procedures are gentle, safe, non-invasive, and keep the pelvis and spine in correct position. This allows your baby more space to move and to grow and helps to keep you poised and balanced. As birth approaches, your baby will be better able to move into the ideal position for birth—creating an environment for an easier, safer delivery.

I have seen chiropractic care work effectively for my daughter, throughout her pregnancy and particularly for the birthing. Consider visiting a prenatal chiropractor especially if you are experiencing physical discomfort during your pregnancy.

A comfortable Mom is a happier Mom.

A final word about honoring your body: After you have your baby, it makes it so much easier to return to a pre-pregnancy shape and size – or even better!

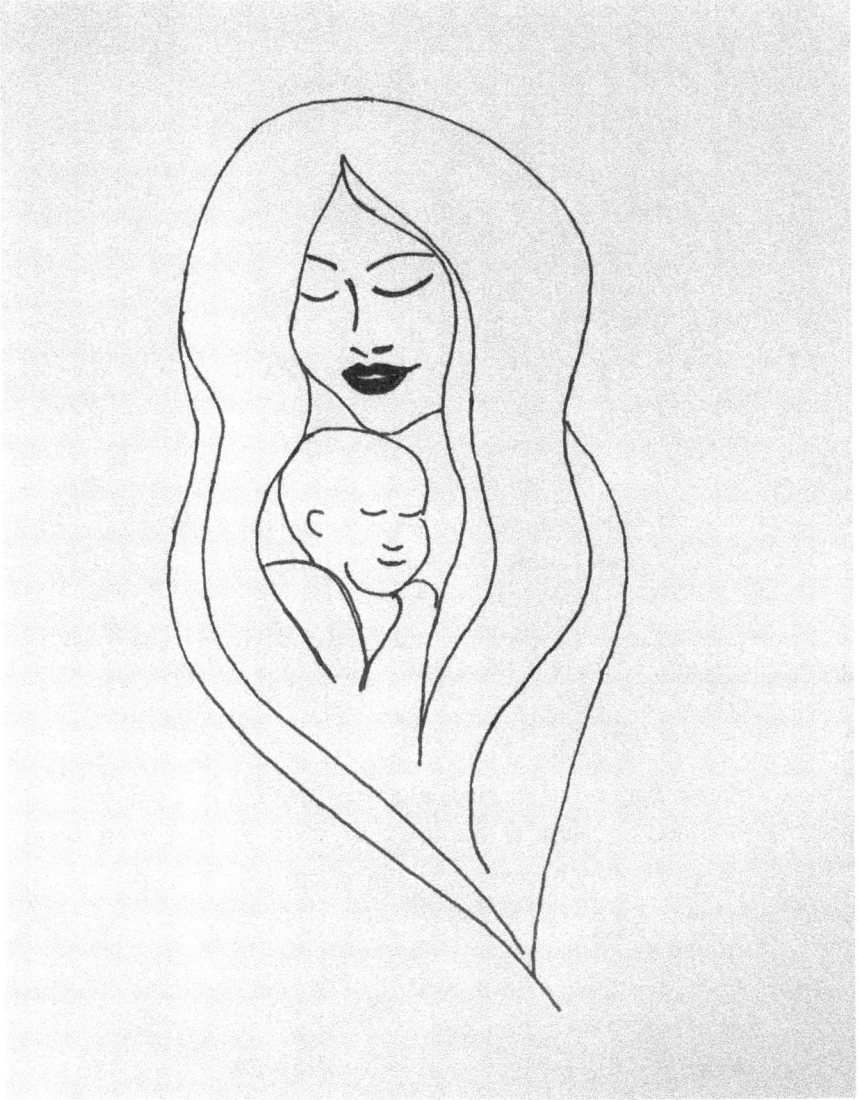

Chapter 4
The Magic Of Mental Power

*"What the mind can conceive, and the heart
can believe, the body can achieve."*

Our minds control our emotions, our bodies, and our behavior. When we train our minds, we increase its power to help achieve our goals and desires. What specifically are your goals and desires right now?

- Do you want to experience a joyful, fulfilling pregnancy?
- Do you really wish to achieve a superior birthing performance that is natural, safe, pain-free, and comfortable?
- Do you want a normal, healthy, and happy baby?
- Can you see yourself achieving these goals?
- Are you willing to commit the time and effort needed to prepare yourself to achieve these goals?
- Do these goals *excite* you and *move you to action?*

Answering "yes" to these questions puts you on the path to success; so let us begin.

Your mental training will cover the following areas:

1. Improving your concentration and focus of attention
2. Monitoring and managing your thoughts

3. **Developing and utilizing imaging and creative visualization skills**
4. **Learning self-hypnosis and hypno-meditation.**

The mental skills outlined above will enable you to attain a state of mind which blocks the negative thoughts and physical discomfort that interfere with your focus on the birthing process and your enjoyment of this experience.

First, let me remind you of the unlimited power of that amazing bio-computer, the brain. Actually, you have two sides of your brain: the left and the right hemispheres. The left brain is dominant in the use of logic, words, numbers, sequence, analysis, lists and linearity. The right brain is dominant in such areas as rhythm, imagination, intuition, daydreaming, color, gestalt (whole picture) and spatial awareness. In our civilized world, greater emphasis and importance is placed on the development of left-brain skills, leaving right-brain skills underdeveloped and underutilized. Tony Buzan, in his book *Use Your Head,* tells us that by stimulating and utilizing the skills of both sides of the brain we can learn to do anything and do it with excellence.

Pregnancy and birthing are essentially multi-sensory, holistic experiences involving every aspect of our total being–physical, mental, emotional, and spiritual. The brain controls the functioning of all these areas. We therefore need the integrated use of the mental skills of both sides of the brain to better enable us to develop these capabilities and to achieve our goals.

All the exercises in this chapter are designed to develop the mental skills of both sides of your brain, so that you can utilize "whole brain" functioning. Mental gymnastics is just as important as physical exercise. This will strengthen your personal power during pregnancy and birthing as well as in all other areas of your life.

1. <u>Improving Your Concentration and Focus Of Attention</u>

The success of any of our endeavors is determined essentially by our ability to maintain a focus of attention to the task at hand. This requires a high level of mental discipline. A mother-to-be will be required to focus her attention on the specific task of birthing her baby and not be disturbed by personal discomfort or external distractions. Here are 2 exercises that will help you to strengthen this ability.

EXERCISE 1: Focusing Your Attention

You can begin by simply focusing your attention on a flower. Keep your eyes glued to the flower of your choice. Hold it about 18 inches away from you and allow yourself to observe it closely. Notice the texture, size, shape, and color of its petals. Look deeply at its center. Contemplate its nature. Spend 5-10 minutes in focused attention. If your attention strays when an extraneous thought enters your mind, just let it go and bring your attention gently back to the flower. You can practice this exercise with any small object such as a ball, a fruit, or a pen, or the flame of a lighted candle. Perform this exercise at least once a day or as often as you can. As you increase you power of concentration, you will find that it becomes easier for you to relax any part of your body at will and maintain an inner calm.

EXERCISE 2: Brain Fitness Exercise

This is a very effective exercise for improving your overall brain performance. It will also give you greater control of your thoughts, improve your mental alertness, your memory, and increase your peripheral vision and speed reading ability.

- Sit on a chair with your back straight and your feet flat on the floor. Allow your hands to rest unclasped on your lap
- Focus on a small spot at a 45 degree angle. Keep your eyes glued to that spot. You may blink if necessary, but try not to shift your eyes.
- Identify:
  - o 3 things you see
  - o 3 things you hear
  - o 3 things you feel

- Identify:
    - o 2 new things you see
    - o 2 new things you hear
    - o 2 new things you feel
- Identify:
    - o 1 new thing you see
    - o 1 new thing you hear
    - o 1 new thing you feel
- Close your eyes and breathe slowly and deeply three times
- Say with conviction:
    "I control my own thoughts.
    I control my own feelings.
    I control my own actions.
    And God is helping me in every way."
- Open your eyes, take a deep breath, and stretch.

This exercise is based on the Betty Erickson Technique for self-hypnosis so you will find that it can also help you to go more quickly and deeply into self-hypnosis or meditation since it prevents wandering thoughts and helps you to focus your mind.

I remember doing an exercise similar to this one (without the breathing, affirmations, and spiritual component) when I first went back to university to do my Masters in Counseling Psychology. I was the oldest student in the class and I felt I had cobwebs on my brain. The other younger students were so quick and alert! I needed to activate my brain functioning to enable me to concentrate for longer periods and to memorize and recall faster and more accurately. I discovered this concentration exercise and it was suggested that I do it once or twice a day. I added the affirmations and I was so motivated that I practiced it 4–5 times a day! I placed post-it stickers all over the house to remind me to do it. I practiced in the bathroom and while watching TV (during advertisements); I practiced it on the patio, in the car (before starting to drive), and at my study desk; I practiced it while sitting, standing, or lying in bed. It was a great way to refresh myself, clear my head, or help me to fall asleep. The good news is that it worked for me. And it can work for you too!

2. <u>Monitoring and Managing Your Thoughts</u>

"A man is what he thinks all day long."
                                        Ralph Waldo Emerson

There is a constant interaction between your thoughts, your feelings, and your actions.

For example: (a) If you ***think*** that someone is coming to harm you, you will ***feel*** fear and hostility towards them, and then as a result you may have to choose aggressive or defensive ***action.*** (fight or take flight):

THOUGHTS→FEELINGS→ACTIONS

(b) If you are doing charitable work (***action***) you can increase your empathy for others (***feeling***) and strengthen the belief (***thought***) that we need to help each other.

ACTION→FEELINGS→THOUGHTS

(c) If you ***feel*** anger towards someone you will probably think negative ***thoughts*** about that person which can trigger a defensive or aggressive ***reaction***.

FEELINGS→THOUGHTS→ACTIONS

So we really need to manage our thoughts, our feelings and our actions. Let us now focus on managing the quality of our thoughts which can be the most difficult to control. Scientific research has shown that the quality of our thoughts affects the chemistry in our bodies.

Negative thoughts change the frequency of the neurotransmitters in the brain and give rise to chemicals such as cortisol and adrenaline that affects our bodily functions and can lead to aggressive or depressed behavior. These negative thoughts become limiting paradigms and prevent us from developing our fullest potential and enjoying the fullness of life.

Positive thoughts also affect the frequency of the neurotransmitters in the brain which secrete other chemicals such as oxytocin and endorphins that lift the spirit, energize the body, and produce positive behavior. So obviously we must learn to think more positive thoughts. That is easier said that done, but with effort it can be done. There are several ways of managing the thoughts that flow through our minds. The key to this is to get into the habit of being sufficiently aware of our thoughts so that we can constantly monitor them. The positive ones we can foster. The negatives ones we can cancel out and replace with more positive ones. Begin with these two effective exercises.

EXERCISE 1: Cancelling Negative Thoughts

Let us look at some negative thoughts, general ones as well as those specific to pregnancy and birthing.

1. List your negative thoughts in the left hand column of the following table.
2. Cancel out each of these negative thoughts, saying to yourself emphatically *"Cancel that!"* and putting an **X** over all of the negatives.
3. Transform each negative thought into a positive, empowering thought and write it in the column on the right. Here are some guidelines for creating empowering thoughts:

- Keep it simple.
- Keep it short.
- Keep it positive.
- Keep it in present tense.
- Use these positive thoughts as affirmations.

This is how it goes: *"Birthing will be painful."* (negative thought) Say strongly, *"Cancel that!"* or *"Delete! Delete!"* Then affirm: *"Birthing is comfortable and natural."*

I have given you some examples of how you can transform these negatives thoughts into empowering thoughts. Complete the transformation of any other negative thoughts that you may have on your list.

KEEPING IT POSITIVE!

CANCEL THESE Negative, Limiting Thoughts	*USE THESE AS* *AFFIRMATIONS* Positive, Empowering Thoughts
1. Birthing will be painful.	**Birthing is comfort-able and natural.**
2. I dread those painful contractions.	**I welcome each surge of divine energy. My birth channel is opening.**
3. Suppose something goes wrong.	**God is in charge. I can manage whatever happens. My birthing team is capable.**
4. I can't do it.	**I can do it. I have the ability to do it. I am capable and well prepared. God is helping me.**
5. Labor can be long.	**The birthing process takes time.**
6. _____	_____
7. _____	_____
8. _____	_____

Here are some other examples that may take place in your everyday functioning:

1. A speeding vehicle swerves in front of the car you are driving and you think, *What a stupid fool!* Immediately say to yourself *"Cancel*

that!" Then add a positive: *"He is in a hurry to meet his Creator. God Bless."*

2. A person close to you (spouse, friend) snaps at you for no apparent reason and you immediately think *"He/she is trying to hurt me."* Say*," Cancel that!"* and replace with *"He/she is having a personal problem and is not dealing with it properly. I will give them space and try to help later."*

3. You forget to practice some of your preparation exercises. You think *"I am never going to be able to do this right* or *I am not capable of achieving my goal."* Say, *"Delete! Delete! Cancel! Cancel!"* Then add: *"I can try harder"* or *"I will do all my exercises today and regularly from now on. I want to succeed, I can succeed, and I will succeed!"* Strengthen your belief in yourself, strengthen your will, and strengthen your action.

EXERCISE 2: Affirmations

The great Roman philosopher Marcus Aurelius asserted, ***"Our life is what our thoughts make it."*** Affirmations are positive statements that we can program to become recurring thoughts. Remember that our minds are like computers—we get out of them what we put into them. So, we all need to take charge of our minds by filling them with empowering, positive thoughts.

If we keep thinking that birthing is going to be agonizing and painful, then we will resign ourselves to making this our experience and it likely will be so. This is the law of the self-fulfilling prophecy. On the other hand, if we choose to think that pregnancy and birthing can be beautiful, natural experiences, then they will likely be so. As Shakti Gawain says*, **"It is these thought forms that ultimately attract and create everything that happens to us."*** This is not a totally passive occurrence because a strong thought propels us to do whatever we need to do to make that thought a reality.

Here are some other examples of affirmations that you can use. Choose the ones that are appropriate and resonate for you:

- I am a birthing goddess.

- God is in charge.
- Divine light and energy is flowing through me.
- I am relaxed and centered.
- I am capable and well-prepared.
- I love and appreciate myself as I am.
- Everything is working for my good.
- I can do all things through God who empowers me.

How to Make Affirmations Work for You

Affirmations become powerful and effective when we use them regularly and thoughtfully.

- Keep them recurring as 'inner self-talk' while walking, showering, driving, or at any other appropriate time.
- Whisper them to yourself as if you are telling yourself a secret.
- Speak them aloud privately or with someone who will support and validate you.
- Write them in notebooks or on post-it notes and stick them in places that you can easily see them as a reminder (e.g. mirrors, bathroom, and car).
- Repeat them to yourself while doing self-hypnosis as a powerful post-hypnotic suggestion. This helps affirmations to become ingrained in our subconscious mind.
- Say them as part of your prayer to God as you surrender yourself. Ask and you shall receive.
- Use them as a mantra at the beginning and again at the end of your meditation when your mind is most open and receptive.
- Repeat them to yourself just before going to sleep and as soon as you awaken.
- Record them on audio tape and play the tape back whenever you can: for example in the car.

I have offered you here quite a number of ways to use your affirmations. Try all of them and choose the ones that are most effective for you. Take charge of your mind! Watch yourself talk. Cancel-out the negatives before they run away with your mind and affect your feelings. Then immediately replace the negatives with strong, positive thoughts. Act decisively and recover control of your own God-given bio-computer!

3. <u>Developing and Utilizing Imaging and Creative Visualization</u>

"Knowledge is limited; imagination encompasses the world"
Albert Einstein.

To image is to create a mental picture using the power of imagination. People think in visual images before they think in words. There is power in your mental pictures and, as you know, a picture is worth a thousand words. It becomes a virtual reality—a blueprint. The stronger the blueprint, the more likely you are able to produce the responses that will transform that blueprint into a reality.

Mastering the art of imaging will benefit you throughout your life. It is a fundamental life skill that is being developed and utilized in every area that calls for superior performance. Professional sportsmen use it with great success visualizing and mentally rehearsing their every move to perfect their performance. In medicine, it is used to help patients to relax and heal more quickly. Cancer patients are taught to use imagery effectively to visualize the cancer cells being destroyed. It is now being used in business, education, psychotherapy, show business and for personal development. Imaging is a powerful right brain capability. Anything that was ever created by man was created twice: First as an image in the mind and second, as an expression produced in reality. Such is the potential power of imaging.

Right now you will be using this skill to enhance your childbearing experience. Following are some of the ways in which imaging will help you throughout your pregnancy and during birthing. As you can see, they are numerous and invaluable.

Benefits of Imaging

- It increases your level of confidence and helps you to embrace your role as a Birthing Goddess.
- It helps you to plan and manage effectively your pregnancy, birthing, and transition to parenthood.
- It reduces or eliminates anxieties and fears associated with childbirth.
- It motivates you to action and helps you to enjoy the process of pregnancy and birthing.
- It helps you to break and destroy the "Fear-Tension-Pain" cycle identified by Dr. Grantly Dick-Read in his book *childbirth without fear.*
- It strengthens your intuitive ability and synchronizes your mind, body and spirit.
- It strengthens your mental power and discipline.
- It improves and deepens your self-hypnosis and meditation.
- It strengthens the bond between you and your baby.
- It increases your awareness of your own needs as well as your baby's needs.
- It gives you greater power and control throughout the childbirth process.
- It increases the likelihood of a shorter labor.
- It improves your ability to relax and surrender totally during the birthing process, thus reducing discomfort during delivery and the chance of lacerations during birth.
- It reduces post-partum blues and helps you to more easily maintain your balance after the birth of your baby.

The following exercises will improve your imaging skills as well as your self-confidence. You will then be able to say with increased assurance, *"I can and I will experience a natural, pain free birthing."*

EXERCISE 1: **Accessing your Personal Power through your Positive Experiences**

A. Make a list of some of the positive experiences that you have had in your life. Think of times when you were **relaxed** and really **enjoying** what you were doing, e.g. at the beach, flying a kite, your wedding day, partying, a sexual experience.

List at least **10 joyful experiences**. This is **List A**.

B. Now focus on things you do really well. Things you **feel confident** doing. Things that you did successfully, such as baking a great cake, organizing an event, passing an exam, getting a promotion, winning a competition, meeting a deadline, completing a project, sewing a skirt, planting a garden, or decorating your home.

List at least **10 of your achievements.** This is **List B**.

1. Tick off 3 positive experiences in list A and 3 in List B that are most powerful and vivid in your memory.
2. Relate 3 of these incidents (1from List A and 2from List B) to a good listener with as many details as possible, using the senses of seeing, hearing, feeling, tasting, and smelling if they apply. This will help you to **refresh your memory and stimulate images** in your brain.
3. Now sit in a comfortable position and ensure that you will not be disturbed. Close your eyes, breathe deeply, and relax.
4. Refresh your memory of the positive experience you chose from **list A**. Allow your mind to take you back to this experience that you recently talked about. Relive it fully with your eyes closed:
   i. Look around at your surroundings. Try to recall all that you **SEE:** people and things. What were you wearing? See the colors. Look up, look down and around. Get as clear a picture as you can.

ii. Recall what you **HEAR.** Listen closely to all the background sounds, voices, noises.

iii. Recall what you **FEEL** – Are you hot? Cold? Tired? What are your emotional feelings: happy, energized, relieved, relaxed, fulfilled, grateful, confident?

iv. Relive this experience as fully as you can and notice how well you can **recapture the emotions** connected with this experience. After a few moments of full enjoyment, you can open your eyes and clear your vision.

v. Now in the same way, relive the experiences of the two positive accomplishments you chose from **List B.**

What you are doing here is using imagery to re-access and strengthen your **ability to relax**, to **enjoy yourself,** to **motivate yourself** to action, to **keep your focus,** and to **feel successful** and **confident** – all the inner competencies you need to achieve your goal of a natural, pain-free birthing experience.

EXERCISE 2: Anchoring Your Inner Power

Now I will introduce you to Anchoring which is a very simple technique from Neuro-Linguistic Programming. This anchoring technique will help you to 'hold on' to your inner competencies so that you can use them during your birthing experience.

Anchoring is based on a natural phenomenon of human experience. It is the process by which certain mind states, feelings and responses are associated with an anchor. The anchor (or trigger) can be something you hear, smell, see, taste, or touch, or a combination of these. For instance, a song you hear will trigger certain memories and feelings. So too can the smell of pumpkin pie, or the sight of an altar, or the taste of a particular fruit. Many of these anchors are powerful and work automatically.

Anchors can also be consciously established with a specific trigger so that particular feelings or responses may be quickly re-experienced when we need them. This is what we will do now.

Anchoring Exercise

For this exercise, the external anchor will be touch. Here are some examples of touch anchors: pressing your hand on a certain spot on your body, pressing the tips of your thumb and forefinger together of either hand, or clasping your hands. Choose the one that is most comfortable for you.

The mind states and feelings that we will anchor are **Confidence, Calmness, Relaxation, Focus of Attention, Self-Control, and Enjoyment** – in other words, some of your own inner competencies that you can access. Focus on **recapturing the mind states and feelings.**

1) You will be using the 3 positive experiences you chose from both List A and B in the previous exercise. You are now going to anchor the **feelings** you experienced when reliving these occasions to your own special touch.

2) Sit comfortably in a place where you will not be disturbed for a few minutes.

3) Practice your touch so that you can do it in **exactly the same way each time, with the same pressure.**

4) Release your touch, close your eyes, and allow your mind to go to Positive Experience No.1. Relive it in the greatest detail. Visualize it as clearly as you can. If you cannot 'see' it clearly, then sense it or feel it so that you can recapture the **feelings** you experienced.

5) Try to **intensify those feelings** and when the desired mind states get to a high point, then **anchor them with your touch**. Keep holding your touch. Release your touch as soon as you find that the feelings are beginning to fade (30 sec – 1 min). You only want to anchor the high point – not fading feelings.

   Then open your eyes and clear your vision for 1-2 minutes.

6) Close your eyes again and allow your mind to go to Positive Experience No.2. Relive it fully. Activate all of your senses— what you see, hear, feel, and smell. Breathe deeply to intensify

your internal power. Capture the **feelings** of the experience by anchoring it with your special touch. As the feelings start to diminish, release your touch, open your eyes and clear your vision for 1-2 minutes.

7) Now go on to Positive experience No.3. Relive it fully until you experience the feelings associated with it. Intensify the feelings and anchor them again with your special touch. Enjoy! When your feelings start to fade, release your touch, open you eyes, breathe deeply, and stretch.

8) Testing time: Take a few minutes, walk around and then settle yourself comfortably again. Close your eyes and now activate your anchor with your special touch. Notice how successful you are in reaccessing your desired feelings. **Congratulations!**

Now you need to continue building up the strength of your trigger by anchoring at least 15-20 positive experiences. You can do that by reliving and anchoring 3 positive experiences from lists A and B each day. You will find that after you have done that, your trigger will become automatic and powerful. You will be using this technique as part of your creative visualization exercises to make them even more effective.

Creative Visualization

We all daydream. We relive experiences of the past as we did in the anchoring exercise. We also visualize the dreams we would like to come true in the future. These visualizations affect how we feel as well as how we behave. In her book *Creative Visualization,* Shakti Gawain explains it this way:

> *"The purpose of Creative Visualization is:*
> *To connect us with our beingness*
> *To help us focus and facilitate our doingness*
> *To increase and expand our havingness."*

She explains that you must first *be* who you really are; then *do* what you need to do in order to *have* what you want. Creative visualization can connect you to your true nature of *being* a Birthing Goddess. Then you can *do* your birthing normally, naturally, comfortably, and joyfully and *have* an expanded family that adds new life to our world.

There are many books written which contain creative visualization exercises for improving and developing our abilities to perform better. Some of these books focus mainly on visualizations that are specific to childbirth preparation. You will find a few of them listed at the end of this chapter.

In using the technique of creative visualization, you use the day-dream habit in a more controlled, positive, and dynamic manner. You can also add soothing background music to enhance your experience. I offer you here some of the visualization techniques that I find most beautiful and effective.

EXERCISE 1: Your Spiritual Sanctuary – Your Own Special Place

We all have within our subconscious mind, in our dream world, a private place where we feel safe, secure, and totally comfortable This is a place where we can totally relax, where we can be truly free to be who we are and experience unconditional love for ourselves; a place where we can feel divine energies embracing us, protecting us, and nurturing us; a place of perfect safety, peace and joy; a place where we can experience the presence of our Divine Creator. We can call this special place our Spiritual Sanctuary.

Begin with the preparatory Steps 1 to 4:

1) Sit or lie comfortably in a <u>quiet place.</u>
2) Focus on your <u>breath</u>. Practice your abdominal breathing. Breathe deeply and slowly, following the breath in and following the breath out.
3) Now focus on <u>relaxing your body</u>. You can use the Progressive Relaxation Exercise in Chapter 1 or you can use this simplified version: Begin from the top of your head moving slowly down to your toes, or begin from your toes and move gradually throughout your body to the top of your head.

4) <u>Deepen your relaxation</u> by counting down from 5 to 1 or from 10 to 1, feeling yourself getting more deeply relaxed as you breathe out on every count.

5) Now allow your mind to take you to your <u>Spiritual Sanctuary</u>, the place where you feel completely safe, secure, and at peace; a place where nothing can hurt you or harm you — where you feel God's love protecting you – a beautiful place: beside the sea, in a meadow, a garden, your favorite room, on a mountain top, or on a cloud. Relax and allow your mind to float you into your sanctuary.

6) <u>Explore and enhance your sanctuary</u>. Take your time. Notice what you see, the sounds you hear, the scents you smell, the emotions you feel. Rearrange or add whatever will make your sanctuary even more comfortable. You may add your favorite music or fragrance or color. This is your own special inner place. Feel free to allow your creative mind to improve your sanctuary in any way you wish so that you can feel totally comfortable, safe, secure, and peaceful.

7) <u>Sit or lie comfortably</u> in your sanctuary. Close your eyes and allow yourself to enjoy fully the perfect tranquility, comfort, and safety of your own personal inner space.

8) Whenever you are ready to <u>return</u> to the outside world, you can take a deep breath, count slowly from 1 to 5 and open your eyes feeling rested and renewed.

Practice this visualization as often as you wish. You will find that after a few practice sessions, it will become easier and easier to do, as well as more and more vivid and effective. You can then use your inner Spiritual Sanctuary as a place to retreat whenever you feel the need to focus within yourself and to relax your body and mind. Use it throughout your pregnancy so that you will be able to use it readily during labor as the need to rest, relax, and keep an inner focus is essential at that time.

This Spiritual Sanctuary Exercise can also be integrated into other visualizations, self-hypnosis, and meditation to become even more powerful and helpful during delivery.

EXERCISE 2: Bonding with Your Baby

Begin with the preparatory Steps 1 to 4:

1) Sit or lie comfortably in a <u>quiet place</u> where you will not be disturbed.
2) Focus on your <u>breath.</u> Breathe slowly, smoothly, and deeply following the breath in and following the breath out.
3) Now focus on <u>relaxing your body</u>.
4) <u>Deepen your relaxation</u> by counting down from 5 to 1 or from 10 to 1, feeling yourself getting more deeply relaxed as you breathe out on every count.
5) Gently place your hands on your stomach and then move them around slowly and lovingly, caressing your baby. Imagine your baby responding with delight as he/she receives this loving energy. Visualize your baby smiling. Transmit positive thoughts and positive feelings of love, security, peace, joyfulness.
6) Coach your baby: *"You remember who you are."* Talk affectionately about your love, what you are doing, the birthing process, and his/her role in the process as part of a divine birthing team. Speak about the family waiting to welcome him/her. Describe the beauty of this world: of nature: e.g. sky, flowers, birds;

    people: e.g. friendships, support, talents;

    positive developments: e.g. technology, science, education.

    You have much to share with your baby. Share a little at each bonding session. LISTEN, SEE, and FEEL your baby's responses.
7) Focus deeply and allow that connection to strengthen as you visualize Divine Light and energy infusing you both and keeping you both connected to a Divine Source. Enjoy that feeling of security and comfort and share it with your baby.
8) When you feel ready to return to the outside world, you can again refocus on your breathing. Count from 1 to 5 very slowly and on the count of 5, open your eyes, take a deep breath, and stretch.
9) Keep remembering that your baby is very connected to you right now and is strongly influenced by both your thoughts and your feelings. At every opportunity, talk affectionately to your baby.

EXERCISE 3: Mental Rehearsal: Using Imagery to Prepare You for Birthing

> *"It's a funny thing about life;*
> *if you refuse to accept anything but the best you very often get it."*
> Somerset Maugham.

The more you rehearse, the stronger the blueprint becomes, and the more likely you are to respond correctly in the midst of delivery. You are training your mind and body to perform in harmony with each other.

BENEFITS

Mental rehearsals help you to:

- Create for yourself a "blue print" of the best possible delivery.
- Rid yourself of self-limiting concepts and behaviors.
- Reduce any undue anxiety before and during birthing.
- Realistically develop the birth plan that is best for you.

Begin with the Preparatory Steps 1 to 4.

1) Sit or lie comfortably in a <u>quiet place</u> where you will not be disturbed.
2) Focus on your <u>breath.</u> Breathe slowly, smoothly, and deeply following your breath in and following the breath out.
3) Gradually, consciously <u>relax every part of your body.</u>
4) <u>Deepen your relaxation</u> by counting down from 5 to 1.
5) Allow your mind to take you into the future where you realize that the birthing process has begun. You are experiencing regular surges of energy. <u>Activate your anchors</u> with your special touch.
6) Experience how you feel and what you do. Mentally rehearse in detail how you would like the birthing to be for you. Use all your senses; see, hear, smell, feel, and taste. You are completely relaxed and comfortable. You are happy that your baby will be born soon and excited that the birthing process has begun. You are fully

prepared for your performance. You feel confident, calm, capable and ready to give of your best.

7) **See** the members of your birthing team around you. See them doing what you want them to do to-support you. **Hear** the music, voices, and sounds around you. **Smell** the fragrance in the air. Your sense of smell is often sharpened. **Feel** the comforting touch of your support team. Go through as many details of your blue print as you can, making it as realistic as possible.

8) **See** and **feel** yourself maintaining your inner focus and yet remaining aware of what is taking place. **Hear** yourself repeat your affirmations. You are breathing comfortably and effectively. **See** yourself welcoming each surge of Divine Energy. **Feel** the tightening of your muscles as they slowly and gently soften and open your cervix. Visualize your cervix as a flower that is gradually opening—each petal gently moving into place, getting ready for your baby to slip through easily. With each surge of energy, you breathe and relax even more deeply. Each surge signals the opening of your passageway through which your baby must journey. Breathe in deeply; breathe out slowly, gradually relaxing your body. Visualize your pelvic muscles gently stretching and opening up. Your cervix is a flower opening into a full bloom to facilitate the birth of your baby. You, your baby, and God are working together as a team to move your baby down and out through your birthing channel.

9) Visualize your baby safely delivered into your arms. Enjoy fully this moment. All is well. You and your baby are both safe and comfortable.

10) Take your time and when you feel ready to return to the outside world, you can again refocus on your breathing. Count from 1 to 5 very slowly and on the count of 5, open your eyes. Take a deep breath and stretch.

Your partner or birthing team member can read the script slowly and softly for you during your practice sessions. There are several beautiful birthing scripts and recordings with accompanying music available for you to use for your mental rehearsal practice. Shop around and try some of them until you find the ones that work best for you. At the end of this chapter, I will list some that are available.

4.Learning Self-Hypnosis and Hypno-Meditation

"It is not enough to have a good mind.
The main thing is to use it well."

Rene Descartes.

There is nothing mystical about hypnosis. In fact, hypnosis is another natural phenomenon that we experience in everyday life. For example, we may drift into a state of self – hypnosis while being engrossed in a movie, listening to music, staring at the burning embers in a fireplace, while watching television or reading an interesting book.

Still, there is a great deal of misinformation and misconception about hypnosis. I only understood the truth about hypnosis when I studied and trained to practice hypnosis, hypnotherapy, and neuro-linguistic programming. I had heard the word 'sleep' being used in many hypnotic inductions by stage hypnotists and in movies, so I thought that hypnosis was about putting yourself to sleep. But that is not so at all.

Hypnosis is totally the opposite of sleep. In sleep, the individual is not conscious or aware of what is taking place and the body may or may not be relaxed. The sleep state will certainly not be helpful to any woman who wishes to participate in the birth of her baby. In a state of hypnosis, the individual is conscious and aware of what is taking place. In addition there is increased concentration and focus of attention, increased relaxation of the body, and increased susceptibility to suggestion. In this state, body and mind are working together harmoniously so that you can enjoy having your baby with the minimum of discomfort. Even though you may sometimes look as if you are asleep when you choose to close your eyes, you can hear, feel, see, smell, and taste. You will have even more control of all your senses and faculties and will be totally aware of what is taking place within you as well as around you. Eye closure is not fundamental to hypnosis. With open eyes you can still enjoy the benefits of being in a hypnotic state.

Benefits of Self-Hypnosis

1. It prepares you to fully experience the joy of a natural, pain free childbirth.

2. It empowers you to manage each stage of your pregnancy and especially the birthing process. You are in control!

3. It enables you to harness the combined power of both your conscious and subconscious minds to achieve your goal. You will be aware and fully focused on what you need to do and will be able to communicate positive suggestions directly to your subconscious mind to facilitate a comfortable, easy delivery.

4. It increases the effectiveness of all your other preparation and training techniques:
   - You will be able to relax both your body and mind more quickly, easily, and profoundly.
   - Your visualizations will become more distinct, meaningful, and powerful.
   - Your meditation will become deeper.
   - Your motivation and commitment to succeed will be stronger.
   - Your physical, mental, and emotional proficiency will improve.

5. You will more likely have shorter labors, use less medication, and experience less depression after delivery. (This was validated by a study done by researchers at the University of Wisconsin and published in 1990 in the "Journal of Consulting and Clinical Psychology.")

Understanding More About Self-Hypnosis: How does it work?

Hypnosis makes all these benefits possible because it gives you direct access to the sub-conscious mind which is the seat of our emotions, our imagination, and our memory. In addition, the subconscious controls and regulates our habits and energy, and the involuntary functions of our bodies such as breathing, circulation, and digestion. That is why it is so important to understand how it works and then to harness this God-given power to help us to develop our potential in a positive way.

During our early childhood in our formative years, our uncritical minds are programmed by many garbled assortments of half-truths, false fears, and prejudices which are ingrained in both our conscious and sub-conscious minds. We carry this information into our adult lives and we function on the basis of this programming often without being aware that we are doing so.

Our functioning is determined by the interaction between our conscious and sub-conscious mind.

Our conscious mind is the intellectual, reasoning mind which can logically decide on a course of action. Our sub-conscious mind is our source of energy which puts that decision into action. It is the 'engine room' that supplies the power to the conscious mind and drives it to achieve goals.

The sub-conscious mind automatically controls most of our behavior, our emotions, sensations and habits. It is in essence much more powerful than our conscious minds. That is why when the conscious and sub-conscious do not agree the sub-conscious usually wins out. For instance, most fears are the result of early childhood programming or experiences that become deep-seated in our subconscious, i.e. fear of water, heights, and closed areas. Even though as an adult, you may consciously know that there is nothing to fear, your subconscious mind takes control and you continue to fear and avoid these situations.

If there is any deep-seated fear of childbirth in the sub-conscious, it will surface during birthing and trigger the fear-tension-pain syndrome. These fears may have been lodged during early childhood and reinforced by many years of negative programming that occurred while listening to family, friends, and neighbors tell horror stories of childbirth, or while watching birthing women on television screaming with pain and writhing in agony. The sub-conscious then believes as absolute truth that birthing is inevitably very painful and to be feared.

Therefore, it will not be enough for you to agree with your conscious reasoning mind that, yes, you want to and can birth your baby without pain and that contractions and delivery can be a pleasant, wonderful experience for you. You will also have to reprogram your sub-conscious mind which is the store house of memories where many deep-seated fears related to childbirth may be entrenched.

To achieve natural pain-free childbirth, you must be free of this fear so that both your conscious and sub-conscious minds will work harmoniously together for you to truly enjoy this wondrous experience of birthing.

Hypnosis is one of the the fastest and most effective ways of reprogramming the sub-conscious mind. During hypnosis, the conscious mind is bypassed or inhibited. Powerful and positive suggestions can then go directly to the sub-conscious to cancel out negative programming and to take its place. This new positive programming must then be reinforced daily until it becomes so deeply entrenched that it can generate and release the energy you need to attain you goals. When the goal that your conscious mind sets is in keeping with the goal in the sub-conscious, then success is inevitable. You have the power to direct your sub-conscious mind to work for rather than against you. Hypnobirthing is the term used when self-hypnosis is utilized for achieving a pain-free, natural experience of childbirth.

Experiencing Hypnosis: How does it feel?
Both hypnosis and self-hypnosis feel the same way and they are basically both self-induced states. Hypnosis can take you into various levels of consciousness:

The light, or Alpha level of consciousness, is easily achieved. At this level you will feel pleasantly relaxed and very much as if you are in a day dream. Suggestions and affirmations can be effectively implanted into the sub-conscious mind at this level.

The medium level or the Theta level of consciousness naturally follows with regular practice. At this level you will feel more profoundly relaxed. You arms and legs may feel so light that they may seem to float or are so heavy that they cannot move. You may even lose conscious awareness of parts of your body and be conscious only of your mind.

These sensations are usually very pleasant. Your sub-conscious mind will be even more receptive to suggestions. At this level you will also experience a natural anesthesia which facilitates a pain-free birthing.

The deepest level or Delta level of consciousness is the somnambulistic state where you can open your eyes and still maintain this level of focused awareness. As expected, there is also a heightened susceptibility to suggestions.

During hypnosis, you may move from one level of consciousness to another without even being aware of it. With regular practice you can then chose to go into the level you desire within 30 seconds.

How can I learn self-hypnosis?

From my own experience, I can say that the easiest way to learn self-hypnosis is by allowing an experienced hypnotherapist to get you started. I attempted to learn it on my own by using self-hypnosis recordings. I believe that they were helpful to some extent, but I was not too sure about how deep I was in hypnosis or if I was doing it right. I attended a few sessions with a skilled hypnotherapist who was able to guide me, deepen my level of consciousness, and also implant post hypnotic suggestions into my subconscious to help me improve my self-hypnosis skills. I practiced regularly every day and I was soon able to develop confidence in my ability to use self hypnosis as part of my preparation for pain free birthing and also for my overall personal development. I used it to help me improve my performance in my studies, to manage my emotions of anger and anxiety, and to deal with some of my deep-seated fears.

If you plan to learn self-hypnosis on your own, here are some guidelines to help you get started.

There are six basic components involved in self-hypnosis:

1. Relaxation
2. Concentration
3. Visualization

4. Suggestions
5. Repetition
6. Closure

The following exercises will incorporate these components.

EXERCISE 1: Preparation for Self-Hypnosis

- Allocate 20-30 minutes for each session.
- Choose a quiet place where you will not be disturbed and disconnect all telephones
- Sit comfortably in a straight-backed chair. This prevents you from falling asleep which can happen if you are tired.
- You may then use a recorded self-hypnosis script to begin. (There are many good ones available now and I have listed a few at the end of this chapter).
  OR
- You can also follow these steps:

1. Begin with the Brain Fitness Exercise described earlier (3-2-1). This helps you to focus your attention and to concentrate. Keep your eyes closed and continue.
2. Now focus on your breath, following the breath in and following the breath out. Say to yourself: *"With every breath, I relax even more deeply."*
   Do this at least 5 times. Repetition implants this suggestion gradually into the sub – conscious.
3. Now use the Progressive Relaxation exercise in Chapter 3. Mentally visualize each area of your body, releasing all tension and relaxing completely. Again give this suggestion to your sub-conscious and allow it to work for you: *"With every breath, I release all tension in my body and I relax deeper and deeper into a very restful state."*
4. Visualize yourself floating off into your Special Sanctuary where you feel perfectly safe and secure, and your sub-conscious mind is totally receptive. At this point you can repeat to yourself one or two of your affirmations so that they can become imprinted into you sub-conscious. e.g. *"I enjoy my pregnancy; I enjoy giving birth to my baby; I am a Birthing Goddess; and God is taking care of me and my baby."* Remain in your sanctuary for as long as you wish. At this

time, you may also give yourself this suggestion: *"I go into hypnosis more quickly and easily every time I practice it"*

5. When you are ready, bring yourself to closure and awakening. Say to yourself: *"It is time for me to return to normal consciousness. I will slowly count from one to five, and as I do so I feel energy and consciousness flowing gently through my mind and body. When I get to five, I am wide awake, rested, and refreshed."* Count slowly. Become aware of your breathing and gently start moving your toes, fingers, and body. On the count of five, open your eyes, take a deep breath, stretch, and feel great!

When you first begin self-hypnosis, you may find yourself consciously analyzing and evaluating your experience at every step of the way. That is normal for most people. Perhaps it may even feel awkward. But learning self-hypnosis is like practicing the scales on the piano or learning to drive a car. With regular practice it becomes so easy that it becomes automatic.

As you gain more confidence in your ability to practice self-hypnosis you can then use the following techniques that will help you to go to a deeper level of consciousness where you will experience a natural anesthesia and learn to apply it during the birthing process. At a deeper level, your mind and body will be at a more suggestible state.

Deepening Techniques
Use these techniques after Step 3 or 4 of your self-hypnosis session.

1. THE ELEVATOR. This is a very effective and commonly used technique because it is so easy to use. Imagine that you entered an elevator on the tenth (10) floor and you want to go down to the first (1) floor which will take you to a much deeper state of relaxation and a more beneficial level of consciousness. The first floor can also take you into your personal sanctuary where you always feel totally safe and secure.

   The elevator begins to descend slowly. As you note it passing each floor, you allow yourself to relax more and more and go deeper and deeper into your sub-conscious mind. Speaking slowly and gently you may also give yourself suggestions such as: "*10) ... letting go ... 9) ... more and more relaxed ... 8) ... more and more comfortable ... 7) ... letting go ... 6) ... loose and limp and so relaxed ... 5) ... so calm and peaceful ... 4) ... deeper and deeper ... 3) ... relaxing more and more ... 2) ... letting go ... 1) ... so peaceful and totally comfortable.*"

As the elevator stops on the first floor, the door opens and you walk into your private sanctuary. You feel more relaxed than ever before. You find a place in your sanctuary where you can lie down or sit and enjoy the benefits of this level of consciousness. At this time you can choose to use some of your affirmations as powerful suggestions to your very receptive sub-conscious mind. When you are ready, you can then use Step 5 for Closure and Awakening.

2. GLOVE ANESTHESIA. This can be used very effectively in eliminating discomfort and pain in any particular area of your body during labor and birthing.

There are many variations to this technique, such as imagining that your hand becomes numb from dipping it in ice water or Novocain. You then transfer this numbness to any part of your body simply by placing your hand wherever relief from discomfort is needed.

I particularly like the variation developed by Marie Mongan in her book HypnoBirthing® – The Mongan Method. She suggests that you "imagine that you are putting a soft silver glove on your right hand, a special glove of natural endorphins." These endorphins gradually permeate your hand so that it becomes pleasantly numb. Your hand can then transfer this numbness to any part of your body as you maintain this deep level of relaxation during the actual birthing.

At this level of consciousness, mental rehearsal of the birthing process will also become more effective and powerful as both your conscious and sub-conscious mind will be working in unison to achieve your goal.

Here again, it may be necessary to emphasize that regular practice is absolutely necessary for you to achieve a deeper and more beneficial level of consciousness. Allocate twenty (20) to thirty (30) minutes every day for at least five to six weeks for practice sessions, and then continue more often as you get closer to the birthing time. Whether or not you use the help of recordings or the assistance of a skilled hypnotherapist, learning to do self-hypnosis has several advantages.

- It increases your self esteem and your sense of self mastery.
- It provides you with skills and techniques for self management and promotes independence.
- It gives you the opportunity to progress more rapidly since you can practice as often as you can at home.

I strongly recommend, however, that you do use the assistance of a skilled hypnotherapist to help you overcome any deep seated fears or other negative emotions that you may be experiencing.

Be determined not to get caught in the fear-tension-pain cycle. Self-hypnosis is one of the most effective ways of cancelling that negative sequence and replacing it with a *Love-Relaxation-Comfort Cycle.*

SELF-HELP SUGGESTIONS

There are many articles, images, scripts, exercises, videos and YouTube presentations now available on the Internet that relate to the topics covered in this chapter. Check them out and use the ones that resonate with you. I have listed a few here:

- The importance of Visualisation during pregnancy – Aware
- Guided Visualisation during pregnancy – Fragrant Heart
- Visualise the baby in your womb – Dr. Nitika Sobti
- The Betty Erickson Technique for Self-Hypnosis
- How to hypnotize yourself – Self-Hypnosis – Tipharot
- Self-Hypnosis Instruction, Five excellent techniques – Mandy Bass, mindtosucceed.com

Keep strengthening your mental power!

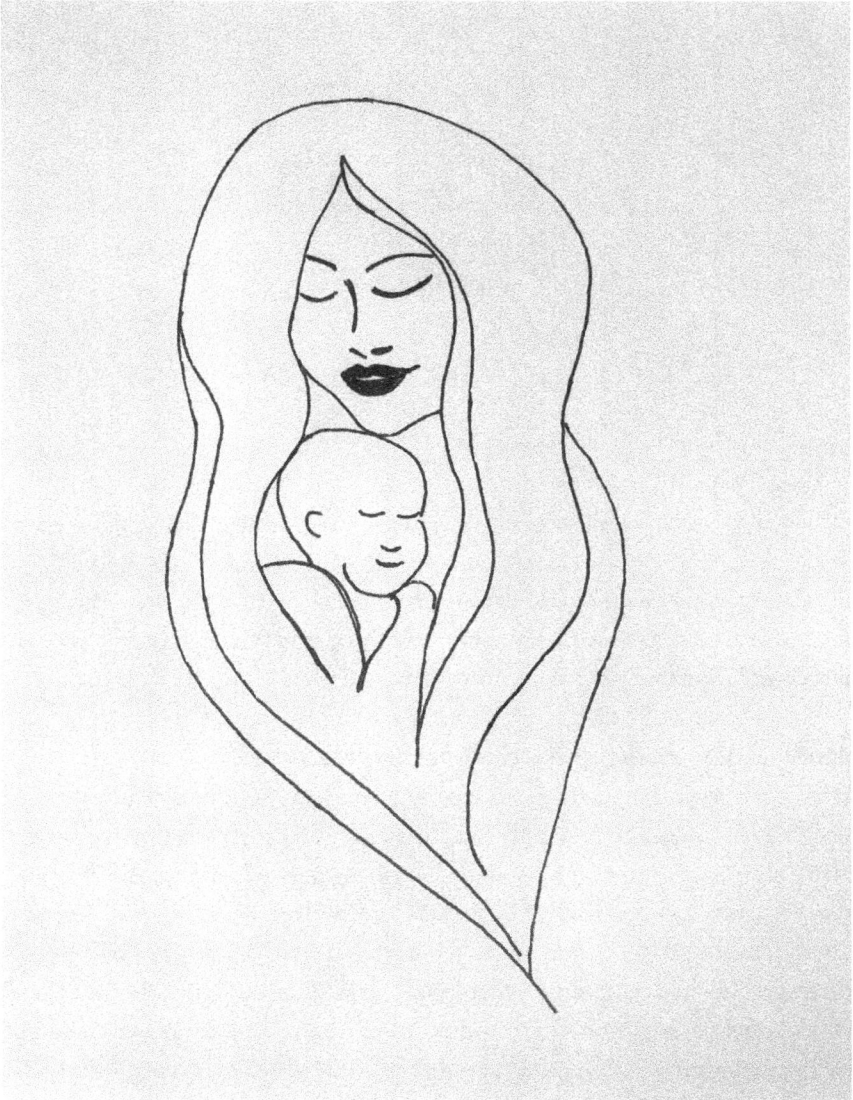

Chapter 5
Your Emotional Garden

Many emotions come into play when you realize that you are pregnant and that there is a baby growing inside your body. What evokes even more powerful emotions is the fact that all your thoughts, feelings and actions will affect the growth of your baby and that you are responsible for the new life within you.

How do you really feel about being pregnant?

For most women, feelings are mixed and can suddenly shift up and down as the pregnancy progresses. Initially you may probably feel joyful and delighted; then you may experience periods of anxiety, fearfulness, worry, and even despair. Or you may at first feel shock, confusion, and apprehension (as I felt for my last pregnancy) and then gradually move on to relief, contentment, acceptance, gratitude, and joy. Be prepared to experience a gamut of emotions, some that you may never have felt before. These emotions can become very intense taking you on a roller coaster ride during pregnancy. So it is vitally important that you can understand and manage them so they do not get out of control.

Many factors contribute to these changing emotions. First of all, remember that emotions are simply a form of **Energy-in-Motion**. We all know that energy cannot be destroyed as proven by Einstein years ago. But it can be transformed to bring positive results, outcomes, and effects. There are a number of energy changes taking place *within* you and *around* you during pregnancy. There are physical, physiological, and psychological changes within you. Shapes are changing, hormone balance is changing, and thoughts are changing. Then, there are the external factors that are constantly changing: your relationship with your partner, your financial situation, your career/job situation, and your general circumstances. These changes can affect your emotions in a positive way or in a negative way. The Choice is yours. You can welcome these changes, manage them for your benefit, and experience more positive emotions, or you can view these changes as 'necessary evils of your condition' and allow yourself to suffer through them while experiencing more negative emotions. Or more likely, you may experience a combination of both which can take you on the "roller-coaster ride." None of us experience only positive or negative emotions. Our emotions may change dramatically or slightly from day to day depending on internal and external changing factors.

Believe it or not, the quality and intensity of the emotions we experience ultimately depend on our attitudes toward pregnancy and toward all the changes it entails. Our attitudes are determined by our mental and emotional programming: our past personal experiences as well as what we learned from other people's experiences, or what we read or saw in movies and on T.V. Remember that much of what we learned about childbirth is based on myths and false beliefs. But we are capable of changing our attitudes by simply seeking out newer scientifically based information to replace outdated negative programming. Today there is a wealth of available factual information about pregnancy, childbirth, and parenting. I wish I had known earlier as much as I know now in these areas. I would certainly have had a more positive attitude throughout my pregnancies and would have handled these experiences better.

With new scientific equipment and methods to observe the internal functioning of the body, researchers are discovering and understanding more and more about how emotions affect the physiology of our bodies. They have found that different emotions trigger different chemicals in the body which regulate the supply of energy and influence body responses and behaviors. For instance, fear activates the sympathetic nervous system which triggers the release of a rush of hormones such as norepinephrine, dopamine, (stress hormones), that create tension in your muscular system. This slows down the supply of blood and oxygen going to your uterus, freezes the cervix and leads to pain during birthing. This, in turn, results in fight, flight or freeze behavior that often calls for pain-relieving drugs and/or medical intervention. On the other hand, trust, contentment, and confidence stimulate the parasympathetic system that generates endorphins that relax the muscles and allow them to work harmoniously to open the birthing channel and facilitate normal, natural, pain free childbirth. It's all about Physics, Chemistry, Biology, and our behaviors. The physics here is of course <u>E</u>nergy in **Motion (Emotion).**

In recent years, there is also more and more evidence that a mother communicates and transfers to her fetus whatever she experiences during pregnancy. Research conducted by the British psychiatrist Dr. Frank Lake, the Austrian psychiatrist Dr. Graham Farrant, and the neuroscientist Dr. Stanislav Grof all corroborate this view. This scientific evidence also validates Hindu mysticism which teaches that the fetus is fed nutritionally, mentally, emotionally and spiritually by the mother's state of consciousness. A pregnant woman continually communicates "messages" to her baby about her own mental, emotional, and spiritual circumstances.

Dr. Frank Lake explains this mechanism in his Report from the Research Department "The catecholamines which convey the 'messages' to do with emotions round the mother's circulation, gearing all her organs and cells to feel joy or sorrow, love or loathing, vitality or exhaustion, pass through the placenta barrier (which to these substances in no barrier) into the fetal blood stream via the umbilical vein." In other words, Emotions are converted in the brain to bio-chemicals that affect both mother and baby.

Psychiatrists, psychologists, and psychotherapists also provide experiential evidence from their own practices which indicates that anxiety, confusion, fear, anger, joy, acceptance, or rejection of pregnancy are all transmitted to the fetus and affect it positively or negatively.

Hypno-therapists have also unearthed this evidence in their practice.

I remember the case of an eleven-year-old boy. His presenting problem was one of extreme fearfulness among other fear-related behaviors. He would not sleep alone in a room with a window. During hypnotherapy sessions, he regressed back to his time in the uterus and experienced extreme fear. When I shared this with his mother, she was totally shocked. She then described an experience she had had when she was about three months pregnant with him. One night, she was awakened suddenly and she saw a burglar coming through her window. She screamed and screamed in fright and became hysterical. The burglar ran and escaped. But that fear had remained with her for a long time afterwards, and she herself lived with that fear even though the windows were subsequently burglar proofed. That fear was transmitted to her unborn son and severely restricted his functioning. Hypnotherapy was successful in removing that fearfulness from both mother and son.

Experiments done as early as in the 1970s by Torsten Wiesel and David Hubel produced scientific evidence indicating that the emotional circuits of a baby's brain are most sensitive to programming during pregnancy. Further research now indicates that sensitivity is heightened in the first trimester! This scientific and empirical evidence makes us realize that we have to be careful about the kinds of emotional seeds that we are implanting in our unborn babies. We have to consider how these seeds affect the growth and personality of our children.

I am sure that each mother wants to have a normal child that is physically healthy, mentally and emotionally intelligent, and spiritually balanced. During pregnancy is then the time to lay that foundation by sowing the seeds of love, peace, contentment, spirituality, confidence, trust, security, and self-esteem – and all the positive and beneficial qualities you want in your child.

I. SOWING THE GOOD SEEDS

This certainly does not mean that you are not to feel angry or frustrated or experience any other negative emotion. Neither does it mean that you are to feel guilty about having negative feelings. Neither does it mean that you must bury or repress your negative feelings.

What it does mean is that first of all you must become skilled at becoming aware of your feelings as they occur. That is, developing the ability to step back slightly from the feeling and monitor it without allowing yourself to become swept away by it. As Daniel Goleman points out in his book *Emotional Intelligence:* "This awareness of emotions is the fundamental emotional competence on which others, such as emotional self-control build." You must first be able to notice: 'I am becoming angry,' or 'this is a strong fear I feel.' Then you are better able to go to the next step and say 'How can I manage this feeling?' or 'What do I need to do to get rid of this feeling.'

So let us go back to the question I asked earlier, "How do you really feel about being pregnant?" Let us examine more deeply the answers to that question. Ask yourself the following:

- Why do I feel that way? What makes me feel that way? Dig deeper.
- What are the thoughts and beliefs that may be underlying my feelings about pregnancy and parenthood?
- Why do I want to have a baby?
- Am I (and my partner) motivated to take the responsibility of bringing and nurturing a new human being into this world?
- Are we well prepared for this journey? What do we need to do to prepare ourselves well?

If your answers stir up any negative feelings and thoughts, then your next step will be to find effective ways to manage or cancel these negatives and replace them with positive feelings. I will be suggesting several ways of doing just that. Try them all and find the ways that are most effective and best suited to you. If your answers are positive, then strengthen and nurture these feelings so that they can help you throughout your pregnancy, birthing, and motherhood. I will also be suggesting ways in which you can foster a positive attitude toward pregnancy and motherhood.

II. MANAGING AND CANCELLING NEGATIVE FEELINGS

Let us begin by dealing with the most crippling and debilitating feeling during pregnancy and birthing – *fear.*

In his classic bestseller on natural childbirth, *childbirth without fear,* Dr. Grantly Dick-Read asserts "The most important contributory cause of pain in otherwise normal labor is fear."

Most women experience some degree of fearfulness during pregnancy. It may be mild in the form of anxiety, concern, or worry, especially if it is the first pregnancy. It may simply be about the fear of the unknown territory that we all have to travel. Or it may be a more chronic fear about the 'horrific pains of childbirth' that has been imprinted on our minds by external influences such as family, friends, media, and religion.

Here are some of the most common fears that may take the form of Anxiety, Dread, Worry or Concern:

A) Fear of the unknown experience ahead, especially if it's a first pregnancy
B) Fear of pain during birthing
C) Fear of something going wrong with you or your baby
D) Fearfulness based on bad personal experiences such as mental, physical/sexual, emotional abuse or a difficult previous pregnancy
E) Anxiety, worry or concern due to external circumstances:
  – Changes in relationship with husband/partner
  – Concern about adequate room/accommodation for baby
  – Worry over finances
  – Anxiety and worry about support available after childbirth
  – Concern about different parenting styles and values
  – Anxiety about greater responsibilities and how they will be shared
  – Concern about suitable birth plan and medical care

At the conscious level, I am sure that you will be able to identify exactly what fears/anxieties you may have concerning pregnancy and birthing. But there may also be fears that have been lodged deeply into your subconscious. People frequently repress painful experiences that can emerge as seemingly irrational fears paralyzing your functioning and robbing you of your enjoyment of life. Bringing these fears to conscious awareness loosens their hold over you and also gives you an opportunity to manage and remove them. There are several ways to get in touch with subconscious fears that can affect your childbirth.

Subconscious fears

Here is a simple and effective technique. It is a form of mental rehearsal. Sit or lie in a comfortable position and close your eyes. Visualize yourself going through your pregnancy–the 1st trimester, the 2nd trimester, the 3rd trimester, and then the birthing experience.

- What do you see?
- What thoughts are going through your mind?
- What do you feel?

Note all of your feelings. Is there anxiety or fear? When do you feel it? How strong is it on a scale of 1 to 10? Then open your eyes and write a few notes about what you saw. What were your thoughts and self-talk? What were your feelings? Did any undue anxiety or fearfulness surface? In what area? How strong were they? Note and describe also your positive feelings.

Acknowledge all your feelings and thoughts, the positive as well as the negative. You can then hold on to the positives and minimize or cancel out the negatives. Now go back to the list of common fears and tick off the ones that affected you most. Add any other concern that came up.

Number in order of importance and intensity the ones you need to address.

Let us now look at ways to eliminate these fears:

A) Fear of the unknown is relatively easy to manage and eliminate. Gaining knowledge and a deeper understanding of what pregnancy involves is the first step. There are many comprehensive books describing all you need to know from up-to-date scientific research on this topic. I have listed a number of books that are a 'must read' that will help you to more fully understand the changes taking place within you so that you will know what to expect. Then there will be fewer surprises or cause for alarm. You can also access a great deal of information on the internet.

Well meaning family and friends may also offer you much information on their personal experiences during pregnancy. Please remember that this information is just the sharing of personal experiences that may or may not be in keeping with your own. Listen and learn and then make a choice of what you want for yourself. For instance: Jane may tell you that she experienced the 'dreaded morning sickness' for six months into her pregnancy and add graphic descriptions of how terrible it was for her. You are in your 3rd month and you experience very slight or no morning sickness at all, and you do not want Jane's experience. The first and immediate thing to do is to mentally cancel out that message from being imprinted in your brain. Say to yourself or out loud, "Cancel! Cancel" or "Delete! Delete!" Then <u>replace</u> the thoughts with positive self-programming. "I feel little or no morning sickness. I feel great every morning. My body is adjusting comfortably to the changes taking place within me."

Then go to the internet and all your books and gain more information on how you can manage, control or 'cure' all morning sickness. Actually I do believe that morning sickness has a strong psychological component – and my own experience validates that belief. I was close to 3 months pregnant when I found out that I was pregnant and did not experience any sign of morning sickness. Instead I felt vitalized and balanced. It was only when I realized that I was indeed pregnant that I experienced my first bout of the 'dreaded morning sickness!' Thankfully, I was able to do a quick recovery from that self-affliction. So check-out up-to-date information on each stage of your pregnancy and manage your own experiences.

Intellectual knowledge builds confidence and helps to banish fears. This knowledge also empowers you to make informed choices regarding all aspects of your pregnancy and birthing. *Be informed*!

B) <u>Fear of Pain During Birthing</u>

In his book *childbirth without fear,* Dr. Grantly Dick-Read has described in detail how fear is the major cause of pain in childbirth. He described it as the Fear–> Tension–> Pain Syndrome.

In the following chart I show the negative effects of fear-based birthing on the mother as well as on the baby. In the adjacent column I then show the positive effects of trust-based birthing on mother and baby.

Negative effects of FEAR-based labor	Positive effects of TRUST-based labor
FEARFUL & APPREHENSIVE	**FEARLESS & TRUSTING**
1. Activates Sympathetic Nervous System (Agitation). Releases stress hormones: norepinephrine and dopamine.	1. **Activates Parasympathetic Nervous System (Tranquility and well being). Encourages release of endorphins and oxytocin.**
2. Defensive fight, flight, or freeze behaviors change the course of natural labor.	2. **Cooperative Trusting behaviors flow with the natural birth process.**
3. Tenses muscles in whole body & mind	3. **Relaxes body and mind.**
4. Shallow breathing, holding breath or irregular jerky breathing	4. **Deep slow rhythmical breathing**
5. Inability to relax and rest between surges	5. **Rests comfortably between surges**
6. Restricts the circulation of Blood to Uterus which becomes hypersensitive and painful	6. **Facilitates normal circulation of blood & oxygen to Uterus.**
7. Lower circular fibers at neck of uterus tighten, and resist dilation – Perineum becomes rigid	7. **Lower circular fibers at neck of uterus dilate – Perineum softens**

8. Vertical & circular muscles in uterus work in opposition to each other, thus causing pain	**8. Birthing muscles work in harmony**
9. Ineffective, painful contractions	**9. Effective contractions.**
10. Prolonged labor	**10. Shorter labor**
11. Birthing muscles tense and result in increased chances of lacerations to mother. Increased birth trauma for baby	**11. Birthing muscles relax & stretch to accommodate baby.**
12. Undue & extreme pressure on baby due to blockage in birth canal.	**12. Baby moves smoothly & easily through open birth canal.**
13. Limits supply of oxygen to baby – fetal distress	**13. Baby receives adequate supply of oxygen.**
14. Possible medical intervention – probable Caesarian delivery	**14. Normal, natural delivery.**
15. Possible physical & psychological negative effects on baby	**15. Healthy, contented baby**
16. Mother feels extreme fatigue during and after birth	**16. Mother has more energy during & after birth.**
17. Partial fulfillment for mother	**17. Happy & totally fulfilled mother**

How then can the fear–tension–pain cycle be effectively eliminated and replaced by the trust—relaxation–comfort cycle?

The most effective way to eliminate this fear is by using a *holistic approach* to childbirth preparation, i.e. by focusing on the balanced development of your physical, mental, emotional, and spiritual capabilities – your total being. A comprehensive training program as described in this book will enable you to achieve the personal power of a Birthing Goddess so that you can truly enjoy your birthing experience.

Here is a summary to remind you of your worthy mission.

EFFECTIVE PREPARATION involves:

- **Physical Training & development – Prepare your body.**
  - Breathing Techniques
  - Relaxation Exercises
  - Strengthening Exercises
  - Balanced Nutrition
- **Mental Preparation – Prepare your mind.**
  - Intellectual Knowledge and Understanding
  - Strengthening Focus of Attention & Concentration
  - Positive Self-Talk – Affirmation
  - Developing & Using Mental Imagery
  - Self-Hypnosis
  - Birth Plan / Pregnancy Training & Birthing Checklist
- **Emotional Preparation – Prepare your feelings.**
  - Eliminate Fear
  - Establish Trust
  - Cancel Negative Feelings
  - Nurture Positive Feelings
  - Strengthen Self-confidence & Self-Esteem
  - Build a Strong Support Team
- **Spiritual Preparation – Strengthen your bond with your Divine Creator.**
  - Prayer
  - Meditation
  - Strengthen Faith

If at any time deeper fears surface or persist, be strong enough to seek out an experienced, qualified hypnotherapist with the expertise to help you eliminate that fear. This saves you time and agony. Hypno-meditation exercises in Chapter 6 can also be used regularly to remove negatives and reinforce positive, peaceful feelings.

C) Fear of Something Going Wrong with You or Your Baby

This is an insidious fear that can be triggered easily by internal or external factors. Thus, you have to be vigilant and deal with it immediately. Keep close contact with your medical caregiver, nurse, or midwife to ensure that your pregnancy is progressing normally. Then relax. Follow your daily routine, strengthen your faith in God, and be sensitive to your body and your intuition. Try to keep a balance. You may use the maxim "Do your best and let God do the rest." That certainly helped me to do what I needed to do and to surrender to God's will. Faith in a Divine Creator (God, Allah, Krishna) definitely banishes fear. So strengthen your faith.

If someone describes a pregnancy that "went wrong", and you find yourself internalizing it and triggering fear in yourself, say to yourself "Cancel, Cancel!" or "Delete, Delete!" and immediately replace the negative thought with an affirmation such as "My baby is perfectly healthy and normal," or "I am enjoying a normal, natural pregnancy. Thank you, God." Of course, if you sense anything unusual, get to your medical caregiver and check it out immediately before fear takes hold.

D) Fear Based on Bad Personal Experiences

These are usually deep-seated fears that may have become chronic if they were repressed and not dealt with therapeutically. I remember an old time saying "Feelings buried alive never die." This is so true.

If you were the victim of any type of abuse, especially sexual abuse, please double check to make sure that feelings of disempowerment, helplessness, anger, resentment or any other negative feelings connected to that abuse are not still buried within you. Sometimes we may think that we have flushed those negative emotions out of our psyche because we have been able to rationalize the experience away. But even though the experience may have taken place a long time ago, the feelings may still remain and affect our functioning. Daniel Goleman explains this phenomena in his book *Emotional Intelligence.* "Our emotions have a mind of their own, one which can hold views quite independently of our rational mind."

I would strongly suggest that if you suffered from any personal abuse, then you should seek counseling, psychotherapy or hypnotherapy to ensure that you no longer harbor negative feelings from that abuse. Inevitably, those negative feelings will surface in one form or another and disempower you and even worse, damage your unborn child. Get rid of them once and for all.

E) Fear, Anxiety, Worry or Concern due to External Circumstances

These issues may not result in full-bloom fears but they can certainly cause anxiety, worry, and concern. Ideally, both parents share in the responsibility to resolve these issues before pregnancy or at the latest within the first trimester of the pregnancy. These issues will not resolve themselves on their own and they are part of the normal package that comes with having a baby. Parents-to-be need to spend quality time honestly, frankly, and realistically discussing these issues.

During discussions practice empathic listening, i.e., paying attention both to the content as well as the emotion expressed. For example if your partner says "How are we going to afford another baby?" Notice that he may also be saying that "We don't have enough money right now to afford another baby," and "I am very anxious and worried about that," and/or "Do you have any ideas?" An empathic response such as "I can see that you are worried about our financial situation" will more likely lead to constructive dialogue and workable solutions. When these discussions are tempered with love, sensitivity, and compassion, mutual agreements and solutions can be reached.

If necessary, seek advice and guidance from an appropriate expert or counselor. The important point here is to resolve these issues early so that pregnancy is not marred by anxiety and uncertainty. It is equally important that you do not inflict these negative emotions on the unborn child.

Managing Anger

Another common negative emotion is anger. Here is what Aristotle had to say about it in the *Nichomachean Ethics*:

Aristotle's Challenge

"Anyone can become angry – that is Easy. But to be angry
with the RIGHT PERSON, to the RIGHT DEGREE,
at the RIGHT TIME, for the RIGHT PURPOSE
And in the RIGHT WAY – that is not easy."

If you are able to rise to this challenge, then you will probably find that your anger has dissipated. Great going!

Anger is definitely one of the emotions that most people find difficult to control because it is normally justified by good reasons. The 'good reasons' are really about needs not being met or perceived unjust treatment in some way. During pregnancy, when big changes are taking place, new needs surface for both would-be parents, so it is easy for these good reasons to trigger feelings of anger. That is to be expected. Anger is not all bad. It brings to the surface internal underlying issues that need to be addressed and corrected. It works as a reminder to resolve existing issues.

Occasional angry moments may not be damaging to mother and baby. It becomes toxic when anger builds on anger and becomes rage fed and fuelled by more anger – provoking thoughts. This rage can consume you or become even more toxic if it is suppressed.

Like all other emotions, anger gives rise to a chemical reaction within the body. Anger stimulates a rush of hormones, such as adrenaline, which increases the heart rate and generates a pulse of strong energy. These angry feelings and negative thoughts are all transmitted to your baby by chemical "messengers" and your baby absorbs whatever you deliver. The longer you allow the anger to remain in you, the more damage you do to yourself and your baby. It is imperative then, that you make every effort to manage your anger and make a quick recovery. Here are some effective ways to manage your anger:

(1) <u>BE AWARE</u> of your own anger signals, e.g. jaw tightening, tension at the back of your neck, biting lips, clenching fist, tears, etc.

(2) Use <u>COOLING DOWN</u> strategies: Anger causes high levels of arousal and strong energy that can last for hours or days. Utilize and burn up that energy in constructive ways and return to a more balanced level:

    a.   Run, Walk briskly, Exercise.

    b.   Breathe slowly and deeply (conscious breathing) refer to Chapter 2.

    c.   Journal. Write down your thoughts and feelings. Research shows a significant decrease in immune cells when hostile thoughts and feelings are suppressed. So express yourself and increase you immunity. Then, it may be a good idea to destroy what you have written. No point holding on to negatives.

    d.   Vent safely. Cry. Talk about it to a friend. Get it off your chest in a safe environment.

    e.   Use appropriate distractions to divert your mind from the problem: Look at T.V. or a movie; Sing; Listen to uplifting music.

(3) Get <u>ANOTHER PERSPECTIVE</u> – from a friend or a knowledgeable or wise person. Sometimes your anger may be based on unrealistic beliefs or on your own underlying unresolved issues. Another perspective can effectively stop your angry train of thought. You can also try to find some humor in the situation. Laugh heartily. It is a good antidote for anger.

(4) Take constructive and assertive action that promotes RECONCILIATION and FORGIVENESS.

    a.   Take responsibility for feelings rather than blame others: Say: "I felt anxious and angry when I didn't hear from you. What happened?"

        This reduces the likelihood of your partner feeling attacked and facilitates a loving discussion and change of behavior to meet your needs.

Avoid aggressive outbursts such as "You make me so angry when you don't call and come home late. You are so inconsiderate." This can be the beginning of a war that only creates more anger and hostility with little chance of a peaceful solution.

b.   Make pragmatic, specific requests such as "Please call me when you are going to be late coming home. I would really appreciate that and would feel comfortable. Thank you."

Avoid vague demands such as, "Pay more attention to my needs!"

Loving words can work wonders. Use this opportunity to nurture a deeper, sweeter relationship between you and your partner. Lovingly and compassionately communicate your feelings and your needs to each other.

Stress

Medical Science has also shown that in cases of extreme stress (physical, mental or emotional), the brain of the fetus is flooded with harmful stress hormones which affect brain development. Remember that "fight or flight" is not an option for a baby in the uterus. Stress, like anger, builds up and can become chronic. Stress is not innately negative. We all need a little in our life to keep us energized. It is only when stress gets too strong for too long a period that it becomes negative and becomes distress. Again be aware of your own distress signals and take steps to alleviate your stress level. Conscious Breathing, Rest, Relaxation, and Meditation can all work effectively.

Depression

Contrary to popular belief, pregnancy does not protect a woman from experiencing depression. Studies show that about 20% of pregnant women *do* get depressed. Mild and occasional depression can be lifted effectively by non-medical intervention with no negative side effects. Psychotherapy, acupuncture, massage, yoga, breathing techniques, exercise, and meditation can all prevent and eliminate depression.

Major depression may need medication. All anti-depressants have side effects and will affect your baby's development, especially in the first trimester. You and your doctor will need to balance carefully the possible risks of medication against the severity of the depression. I would also suggest that you seek a second and third opinion, even if you contemplate taking a natural remedy. There are many options available, so explore and choose the ones most suitable to you with the least risk to you and your baby.

Be open and acknowledge what you are experiencing be it fear, anger, stress, depression, joyfulness, or serenity. Work together with your partner to clear out any toxic emotions so that your home becomes a peaceful sanctuary where you, your family, and your new baby can feel cherished, loved and protected.

III. <u>FOSTERING POSITIVE FEELINGS & EMOTIONS</u>

It is equally important to nurture positive emotions to replace the toxic ones that are removed. Psycho-Neuro-Immunology research that studies the mind-body connection has also validated that positive feelings of relaxation, peace, and happiness drive the brain to release endorphins which enhance a person's sense of security and comfort and restores the immune system. Remember that all emotions experienced by the pregnant mother are transmitted to her unborn baby.

The renowned research scientist in Consciousness Studies, Dr. Stanislav Grof, states: "Positive experiences in the womb and after birth are the closest contacts with the Divine that we can experience during our embryonic life or in infancy."

In essence, a pregnant mother's Positive Emotions will lay the foundation for physical, mental, emotional and spiritual well-being in her baby.

Here are some effective ways to foster positive emotions:

• **Keep a Gratitude Journal**

Unity co-founder Charles Fillmore once wrote, "It has been found by experience that a person increases his blessings by being grateful for what he has."

Scientific research validates this statement and shows that the blessings you receive are not only spiritual, but also physical, mental and emotional. Dr. Christiane Northrup, gynecologist, obstetrician and renowned author on women's health explains that feelings of gratitude and thankfulness effect beneficial physiological changes in your body. Levels of stress hormones decrease, coronary arteries relax, breathing becomes deeper, thus increasing blood supply to your heart and raising the oxygen level of your tissues. In addition there is improved hormonal and immune system balance, more effective brain functioning and a general feeling of well being.

The author of *Simple Abundance,* Sarah Ban Breathnach, says "Gratitude is the most passionate transformative force in the cosmos." For our convenience she has also produced the *Simple Abundance Journal of Gratitude.* This is a beautiful book that will help you to discover and record on a daily basis your many blessings. Her book also includes inspiring quotations and a list of 150 often overlooked blessings as gentle reminders. Your journal is not simply a diary of recorded events. It is a record of your feelings and thoughts of thankfulness for whatever you experience.

I have been using that *Journal of Gratitude* for the past eighteen years and I have noticed that when I journal daily (at the end of each day), I sleep and feel better. It also acts as a positive diary and encourages me to find and document whatever is good in every situation. Sometimes I browse through my journals of the past years, and I get great delight and joy reliving the thankfulness I felt then.

If you are unable to obtain a copy of Sarah Ban Breathnach's *The Simple Abundance Journal of Gratitude,* then make your own Journal with any blank writing book or use a diary and rename it 'My Gratitude Journal.' As you fill your journal with the blessings of each day, you will find yourself enjoying deeper feelings of peace and contentment.

• Be a "Good-Finder"

Focus on finding the good in every situation as well as in every person.

No one is all bad. Everyone has good in them. I remember a poster I once saw: "God does not make junk." People are basically good.

Admittedly, some of us have developed very bad behavior and we may have to look very hard to find the good. But it's there. So keep looking.

This will prevent you from holding on to strong negative feelings toward anyone. Remember your feelings are being transmitted to your baby and I have heard it said that babies can take on the characteristics of someone for whom you hold strong negative feelings. Do you want to take that chance? Find the good that can neutralize some of the negatives you feel. Also, if it is someone close to you, find ways to nurture the positive in them. Show gratitude and praise them for the positive. That will reinforce good behavior and eventually redound to your benefit.

- **Keep a Peaceful Mind**
  - Think peaceful, happy, positive thoughts.
  - Repeat your affirmations and fill your mind with constructive, positive self-talk. Refer to Chapter 5 on Mental Preparation.
  - Meditate regularly everyday.
  - Use your positive visualizations and affirmations during self-hypnosis practice.
  - Pray throughout the day, making a conscious effort to feel the presence of your Divine Creator within you and around you.
  - Listen to soothing and uplifting and joyful music.
  - Look at non-violent movies. A sensitive, strongly visual person can be affected very negatively by internalizing emotions elicited by violent movies.
  - Read uplifting and inspiring books.

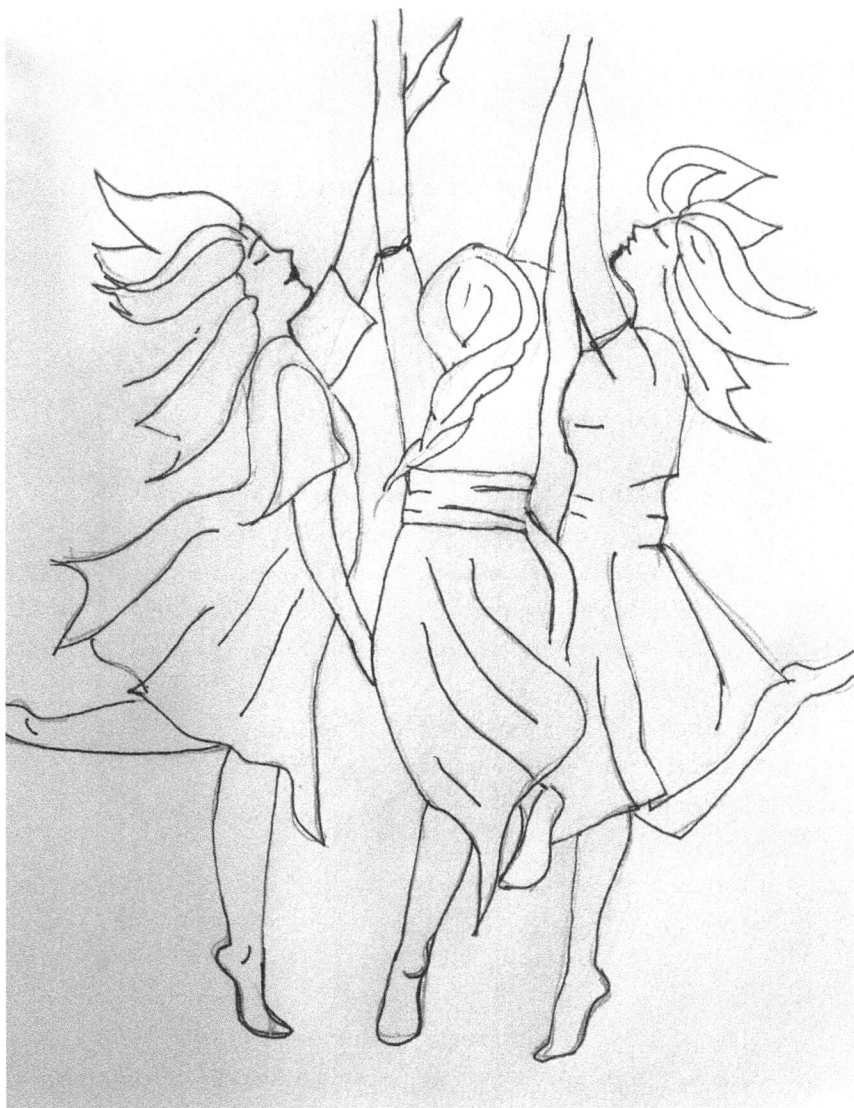

- **Engage In Enjoyable Activities**
  - Find the time to do some of the things that keep your spirit buoy-
    ant and happy, e.g. hobbies, sports, creative crafts, going to the
    beach, dancing.

- Socialize with positive, supportive friends and family. Emotions are infectious!
- Avoid negative people.

• **Allocate Personal Time For Self-Care**
  - Pamper your body.
  - Dress beautifully.
  - Lift your Spirit.
  - Be aware of your feelings.
  - Collect your thoughts – quiet time.
  - Connect deeply with your baby.

• **Create A Welcoming Environment In Your Home**
  - Allow your imagination to inspire you to make appropriate changes in your environment that will keep you focused on joyful thoughts and feelings. The changes do not have to be big changes. Maybe just changing the color of a wall, or adding a plant here or there.
  - Infuse some of your favorite aromas into each room with candles or scented oils: – Lavender, Rose, Ylang ylang.
  - Play soothing music
  - Decorate the baby's corner or room.
  - Encourage other members in your home to join you in your efforts.

Summary

o Manage or eliminate negative emotions quickly before they become chronic. Chronic emotional distress in any form is toxic.

o Resolve problems in a positive fashion – the earlier the better.

o Seek professional help, if necessary.

o Nurture Positive Emotions.

o Sow Good Seeds.

Women do have the opportunity to sow the positive seeds of peace and love in their babies from the beginning of their conception. Women do have the power to change the future of the world by nurturing the hearts and minds of their sons and daughters. Give it your Best!

WOMEN DO HAVE THE POWER AS BIRTHING GODDESSES.

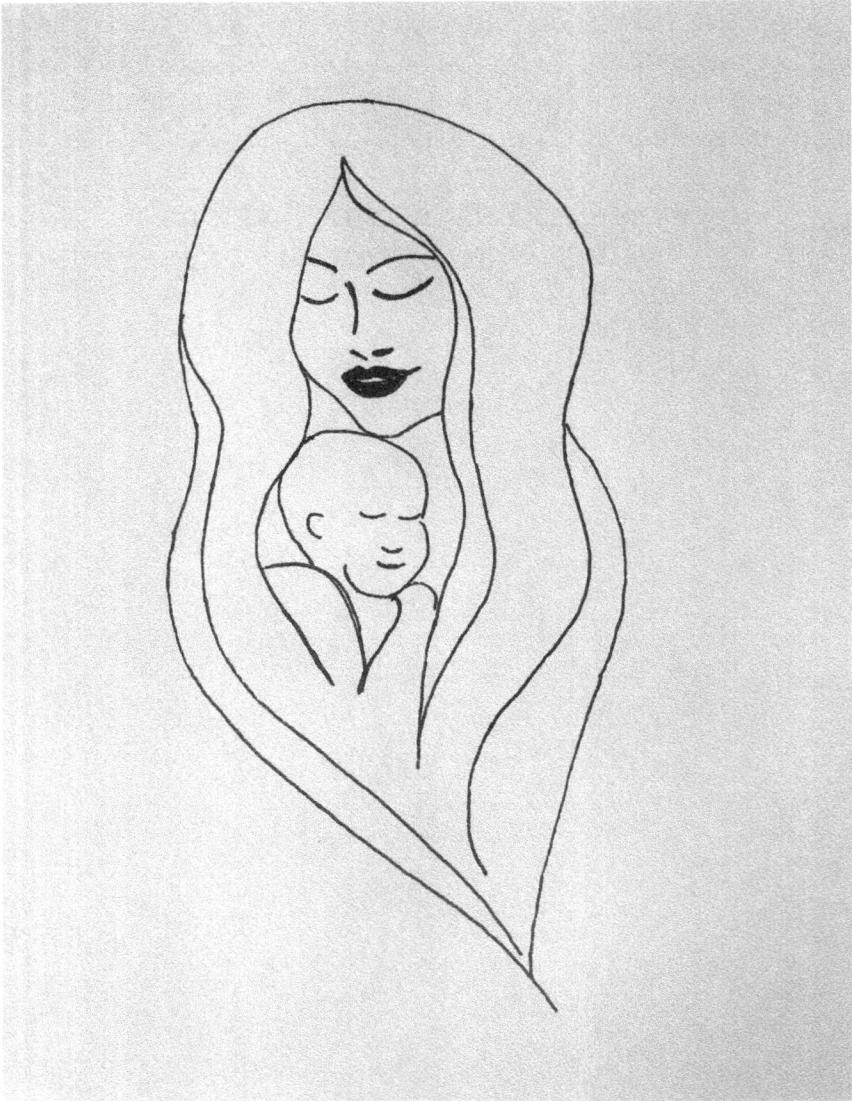

Chapter 6
Nuturing The Spirit

"I believe the choice to become a mother is the choice to become one of the greatest spiritual teachers there is."

Oprah Winfrey

All of our experiences in life are connected to our spiritual growth—and none more so than partnering with our Divine Creator to co-create new life on Earth. The great American psychic, Edgar Cayce states that *"Although ovulation is a law of nature, conception is a law of God."*

The famous obstetrician, Dr. Grantly Dick-Read, asserts: *"Childbirth is not a physical function. The drama of the physical manifestations has blinded its observers to the truth – the birth of a child is the ultimate phenomenon of a series of spiritual experiences, from fantasy to fact and from fact to fruition."* He goes on to say: *"The miracle by which new life is given to us has gained our highest respect, and we have seen in awe, woman pass from the physical to the spiritual comprehension of the magnitude of human love."*

As a pregnant Birthing Goddess we manifest our spiritual connection and our Divine role in procreation. This is another opportunity that life gives us to express the divinity within us by aligning our will with the Divine will.

We can begin by strengthening our prayer power.

Prayer Power

"Prayer is an invitation to God to intervene in our lives."
Abraham Joshua Heschel

Prayer is making a conscious effort to connect with God. When you pray, allow your heart to support your words. Pray with feeling. Pray with passion. Pray with your whole being. This is one time that you don't need a thesaurus. Any heartfelt sincere word will work. Wordless prayer will work also as you humbly surrender your needs and concerns to your God at any time and in any place. That's the beauty and power of prayer.

"More things are wrought by prayer than this world dreams of."
Alfred Lord Tennyson

Begin each day with prayer and gratitude.
Live each day with prayer and gratitude.
End each day with prayer and gratitude.
Make God your personal friend. Talk to Him, commune, and listen. Strengthen that spiritual bond.
Let me share with you a pattern of prayer that works for me:
I always begin by **greeting** God as my dearest friend: "Good morning God:" "Good night, my dearest Friend," or even, "Hi, God!"
Then I **thank** God for as many things that I can think of: my health, a good meal, my family. Next I ask **forgiveness** for any errors or mistakes I made.
Then I **ask** for **help** and **guidance** to correct my shortcomings and for any needs I may have. *"Ask and you will receive."* **(Luke 11:9.)**
You may wish to ask for:

- A happy, normal pregnancy
- A safe, natural, pain free, joyful birth
- A healthy, normal baby
- All the help you need to exercise regularly
- A supportive birthing team

In closing I **surrender** myself and all my concerns to Divine love and mercy, and end with another **prayer of thanksgiving**.

Strengthen your prayer power by praying with others:
"Where two or three are gathered, I am in the midst to bless."
(Mathew 18:20.)

• Pray daily with your husband or partner
• Pray with family members and friends
• Pray with a congregation in church or a prayer group

And always remember to acknowledge with gratitude all the special blessings that you do have.

Meditation

When we pray, we **talk** to God. When we meditate we **listen** to God.

Good communication involves both talking and listening. If we wish to establish a clear strong communication line with God, we will need to practice both prayer and meditation on a daily basis. Talking comes easily for most of us. Listening usually takes greater conscious effort and skill. So too does meditation. Meditation is an invaluable life-skill that can be very beneficial to you throughout your pregnancy and especially during birthing.

There was a time when meditation was cloaked in mysticism, magical symbolism, or religion. Today this is no longer so. Scientific research and innumerable studies on the art and science of meditation provide a deeper and clearer understanding of this practice. There is even scientific equipment and technology that can induce the meditative state and help you to learn to meditate.

In fact, meditation can be learned and practiced by everyone. Because of its wide range of benefits, meditation is now practiced by athletes, actors, scholars, medical practitioners and others for its health benefits as well as for its mental, emotional and spiritual benefits.

While I was pregnant with Athena, I meditated every day, most times every morning and evening for about 20 minutes or more each time, and sometimes for shorter periods (5-10 minutes) before I focused on my studies. This helped me to keep on an 'even keel.' I was better able to free myself from worry and anxiety and to be more receptive to my coursework at the university. My disposition became calmer and more relaxed so that I was better able to manage the 'juggling act' of running the home, paying attention to my children and husband, meeting my course deadlines, and caring for myself and my unborn baby.

I can guarantee that meditation will benefit you in many ways, physically, mentally, emotionally, and spiritually throughout your pregnancy.

General Benefits of Meditation

One of the most wonderful benefits of meditating during pregnancy is that it gives you the opportunity to focus within and to bond with and communicate with your baby in a profound way: body to body, mind to mind, energy to energy, and spirit to spirit. You are then able to establish a positive foundation for your relationship with your baby after birth. Mothering and Nurturing actually begins at conception.

Physical benefits of Meditation:

- It releases you from stress and reduces stress-related problems such as headaches, tension, anxiety, sleeplessness, and fearfulness.
- It lowers your blood pressure.
- It slows the heart rate and increases blood flow.
- It slows breathing down and enables you to use oxygen more efficiently.
- It reduces muscle tension and deepens your level of relaxation.
- It facilitates the release of labor-regulating hormones such as oxytocin.

Mental & Emotional benefits:

- It improves your ability to focus and concentrate.
- It utilizes the right hemisphere of your brain which is associated with intuition, emotion, and imagination.
- It helps you to clarify thoughts, values, ideas, and events.

- It strengthens your own identity as a Birthing Goddess, the essence of your true self.
- It increases your confidence to achieve a safe, comfortable, and joyful birthing experience.
- It decreases the likelihood of depression.
- It gives you greater peace of mind and a calmer disposition while managing daily problems with minimum irritation.
- It gives you greater awareness of how your body operates so that during the actual birthing you can observe your cervix opening and visualize the movement of your baby through your birth channel. As a true Birthing Goddess you will be able to be both an active participant as well as a witness to the power of the birthing process.

Spiritual benefits:

- It strengthens your spiritual connection with your Divine Creator.
- It enables you to access Divine power and to integrate it with your own personal power to provide you with super power.

How to Achieve a Meditative State

Meditation is a process of stilling the mind and resting in the Divine presence. Thinking and self-talk shift to consciously listening which lead to stillness of the mind and communion with God.

There are several ways to achieve a meditative state and many schools of meditation, each focusing on a particular aspect of meditation. However, there are some fundamental components that lead to a meditative state. They are: a) Centering b) Alignment c) Expansion d) Awareness

a) **Centering:** Meditation usually begins with an activity to help you to relax your body and your mind and to center yourself. This may take the form of prayer, conscious breathing, progressive relaxation, repeating a mantra, repetitive movement, focusing on a light or sound, self-hypnosis, a guided meditation or a combination of several of these.

b) **Alignment:** As your conscious mind becomes quieter, you become attuned to your subconscious mind, your inner self. You can then explore and focus within.

c) **Expansion:** Your mind gradually expands as your consciousness embraces the dimensions of inner and outer space. You can then hear the sound of the universe resonating in your ears and throughout every cell of your body.

d) **Awareness:** You become aware of the oneness of the universe and experience the uplifting beauty and comfort of resting in the presence of the Divine Creator.

All this can happen in a few seconds, minutes, and sometimes only after consistent practice sessions. If your mind begins to wander, gently bring it back by refocusing on your breathing, repeating a short affirmation or prayer (like a mantra) or listening for the sound of the universe.

As I said before, there are many styles and paths to meditation. I have been meditating for more than thirty years and I have also practiced several styles of meditation. What I have found is that a combination of techniques can enhance the meditative state. When self-hypnosis is combined with meditation (hypno-meditation) both techniques gain synergistic power and become dynamically effective.

Ormond McGill, an international authority on hypnotism, describes this combination nicely in his book *Hypnotism and Meditation*: "Self hypnosis and meditation are like ice cream and apple pie—the tasting of one makes the other taste better. There is a blending." Hypnotism and meditation are similar in that they both give you access to your subconscious mind, to the alpha, theta, and delta levels of brain functioning. Whereas self-hypnosis is focused on achieving a specific goal, meditation is focused on becoming aware of your true Self – your connection and oneness with the Universe and the Divine.

A guided creative meditation that combines conscious breathing, prayer, affirmation (used as a mantra), relaxation, self-hypnosis and visualization becomes very powerful and effective. Although these techniques may be different and distinct, they are interrelated and each stimulates and facilitates the use of the others. When used together we are combining several aspects of our being: our body, our hearts, our minds, our imagination, our will, and our spirit. When these are synthesized, they become a powerful invocation to our Divine Creator.

Here is a Guided Creative Meditation
The guidelines for practicing meditation are similar to those I suggested for self-hypnosis and creative visualization.

- Allocate 20-30 minutes for each session.
- Choose a quiet place where you will not be disturbed and disconnect all phones.
- Sit comfortably in a straight-backed chair or in the lotus position. (If you are tired and choose to lie in bed you may easily fall asleep).
- Gently close your eyes.
- Have your birthing partner or a friend read this script slowly and softly for you. After a few sessions you may not need the script.

Script:

Focus on your breath. Breathe slowly, smoothly, and deeply, following the breath in and following the breath out..............That's right.

Now take a deep breath........breathing in slowly. Hold it for a second......

Exhale slowly.

Take a second deeper breath. Fill up your lungs now, Feel your diaphragm expanding. Hold.

Exhale very slowly and feel your muscles going limp and loose and so relaxed.

Take a third deep breath........slowly and deeply. Hold for a second....

Exhale slowly......and allow all anxiety and tension to flow out of you, leaving you more relaxed.

Breathe normally now.......and with each breath you become more deeply relaxed and comfortable.

Imagine now that your breath is flowing into your body from the top of your head.

You may see it as a white light or in any colour .Your breath connects you with your Divine Creator. Feel it, see it, sense it ..... this Divine energy is moving in and around the top of your head relaxing and energizing your scalp muscles and gently flowing into your brain helping you to release all concerns and anxieties. Let them go.

Now allow that divine light, that divine breath to flow down into your facial muscles. Feel your face relaxing and going limp and loose .... all the nerves and tiny muscles around your eyelids are easing and letting go like loose rubber bands ...... your jaw and mouth are relaxing too.

Feel that wave of relaxation flowing through your neck muscles, your shoulders, flowing down your arms right to your fingertips.

Relaxation moving easily now through your back, chest, stomach, your cervix, down your thighs, legs, ankles and feet ...... releasing all tension from your body.

With each breath you breathe, you feel more and more relaxed, more and more comfortable, and more deeply at peace.

Let go now and surrender yourself to this beautiful experience.

You are perfectly safe, you are perfectly secure. Nothing can hurt you or harm you.

God's Love is protecting you.

Imagine that you enter an elevator on the tenth (10) floor and you want to go down to the first (1) floor which will take you to a much deeper state of relaxation and a more beneficial level of consciousness. The first floor also takes you into your personal sanctuary where you always feel totally safe and secure. You are in the elevator now. There are seats in the elevator so you can sit and make yourself comfortable.

You allow yourself to relax more and more and go deeper and deeper into your sub-conscious mind as the elevator descends slowly: 10) ... letting go ... 9) ... more and more relaxed ...8) ... more and more comfortable ...7) ... letting go ...6) ... loose and limp and so relaxed ...5) ... so calm and peaceful ...4) ... deeper and deeper ...3) ... relaxing more and more ...2) ... letting go ...1) ... so peaceful and totally comfortable.

As the elevator stops on the first floor, the door opens and you walk into your private sanctuary. You feel more relaxed than ever before. Find a place in your sanctuary where you can lie down or sit and enjoy the benefits of this level of consciousness. You repeat one or two of your affirmations as powerful suggestions to your very receptive sub-conscious mind ....

You say a prayer ....

You feel the Presence of your Divine Creator ....

You surrender your concerns and ask for help ....

You let go and listen in silence to the music of the universe ....

Be still now and enjoy Divine peace for as long as you wish ....

When you are ready to return to full consciousness, you can count slowly from 1 to 5. When you get to 5, you can open your eyes, stretch gently and return to the full consciousness of the room feeling fully refreshed.

End of guided meditation.

Meditation can be even more effective when done with a group of meditators. I usually find it easier to get into a meditative state and find myself more strongly energized when in a group. It is like being refueled. So, seek out a meditation group in which you feel comfortable. Your yoga group or pregnancy classes may also wish to meditate together. Or you and your partner or other members of your family can meet for 30 minute sessions of prayer and meditation every morning or evening.

Once you have gotten into the practice of meditation, you will find that it will become a fundamental part of your daily routine – like brushing your teeth or taking a bath. Prayer and meditation have become part of my morning routine and help me face the day with confidence and calmness.

There are many guided creative meditations available. Some of them combine several of these techniques and are designed specifically for pregnancy and birthing. At the end of this chapter I will suggest some that you may find helpful.

Additional Spiritual Support
Read Uplifting Books

- Spend a few minutes every day reading the scripture that supports your religious belief.
- Read and contemplate uplifting thoughts for each day (keep a pocket size book in your hand bag or office drawer).
- Avoid reading books that are filled with violence and terror.
- Read books that are inspiring and positive.

Listen to Uplifting music

- Soothing classical music, such as Vivaldi, Bach, and Mozart
- Spiritual songs
- Sing-along praise and worship songs
- Lyrical happy music
- Nature sounds – soothing sounds of the ocean or forest

Cultivate Positive relationships

- Build a team of supporters who share your values and spiritual beliefs and can become friends for life.
- Choose the members of your team wisely from among your family, friends, colleagues, neighbors or healthcare professionals.

A supportive team functions as Earth Angels to watch over you and to provide you with appropriate guidance, assistance and encouragement throughout your pregnancy so that your birthing performance can be your best.

Recommended Reading, Meditation CDS and YouTube Presentations

- *Meditations for Pregnancy* by Michelle Leclaire O'Neil. Kansas City, U.S.A. Andrews McMeel Publishing 2004 (book and CD)

- *Hypnobirthing–The Mongan Method* by Marie F. Mongan, Deerfield Beach, Florida Health Communications, Inc. 2005. (book and CD)
- *Hypnotism and Meditation: The Operational Manual for Hypnomeditation* by Ormond McGill published by Westwood publishing Company, 1984, California, USA.
- *Preparing for childbirth – guided imagery exercises to ease labor and delivery* by Dr. Martin L. Rossman (CD).
- *Hypnosis for a joyful pregnancy and pain-free labor and delivery* by Winifred Conkling
- Meditation Techniques for Pregnancy and Labor – Emma Kenny (YouTube)
- Guided Meditation for Childbirth Fear Release – Bailey Gaddis (YouTube)
- Hypnobirthing Meditation for a Peaceful Pregnancy and Beautiful Birth – Aluna Moon (YouTube)
- Hypnobirthing – Guided Meditation – Priscilla Tuft (YouTube)

There are many Guided Meditations for Pregnancy and Hypnobirthing on the Internet. Choose the ones that resonate with you and keep practicing! Enjoy your Pregnancy and Birthing!

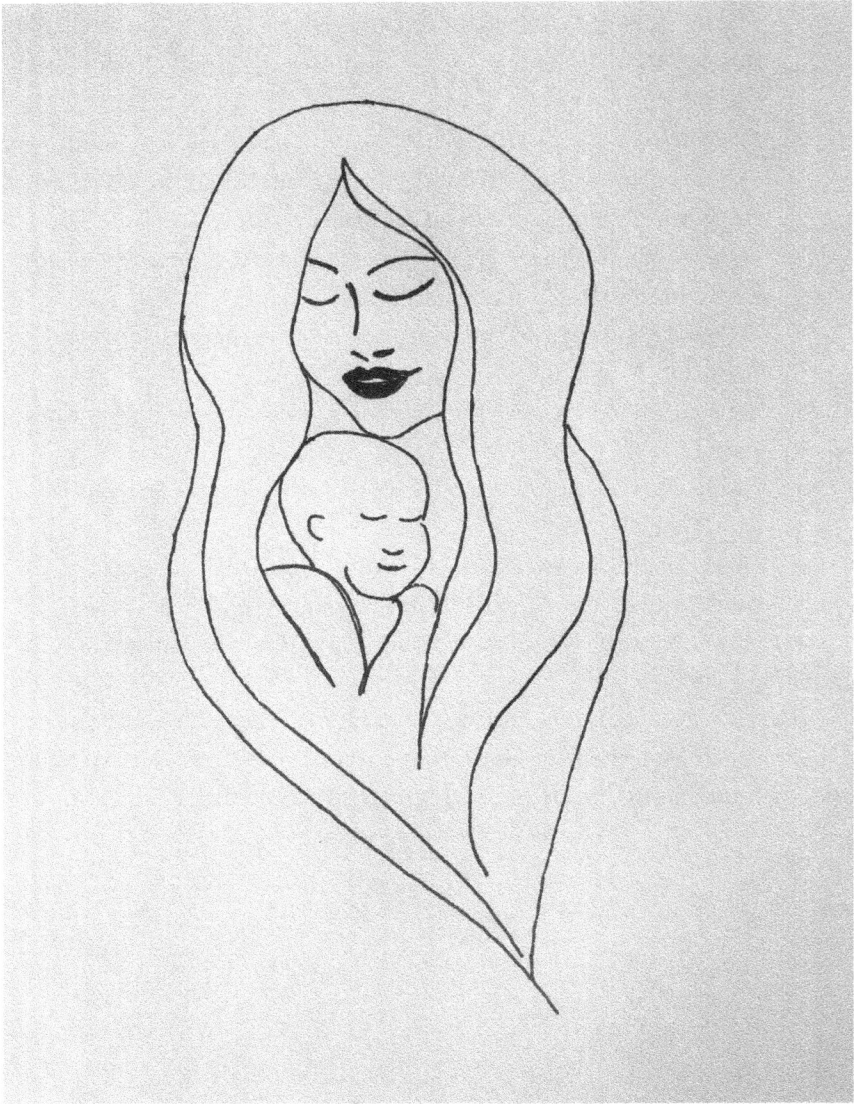

Chapter 7
Dancing With The Goddess – it's a family affair

"Coming together is a beginning, Keeping together is progress, Working together is success."

Henry Ford

Bringing new life into this world begins with the collaboration of a man and a woman. This miraculous unfolding of co-creation commences when the sperm of a man fertilizes the egg of a woman. That embryo of new life contains the DNA of both partners – a joint legacy that together they contribute to the future. Fatherhood and motherhood begins at this point of conception and continues throughout the lifetime of parents.

The responsibility for nurturing and ensuring the healthy growth of this new life lies with *both* partners. Pregnancy, birthing, and parenting are not solely the duties of the woman. In the more enlightened world of today, fathers and partners are encouraged to participate fully in the total process of co-creating new life. This approach brings tremendous long lasting benefits to fathers, mothers, and to the baby. Fathers and partners feel greater satisfaction and fulfillment from being more directly involved in the preparation for birthing and more connected to the baby in the womb of the mother. Women with supportive partners are able to be more accepting of the various stages of pregnancy, a fact that can contribute to an easier and shorter labor and birthing. Of course, the baby first and foremost totally benefits from the combined love and attention of mother, father, and supporters.

It's all about TEAMwork: *"Together Everyone Achieves More"* (Anonymous)

For any team to work well, team members must have a clear understanding of their own roles and responsibilities and be willing and able to support each other to achieve a mutual goal. In this case the pregnant woman plays the leading role as the Birthing Goddess with clear and direct responsibility for the baby within her. Nonetheless, the roles and responsibilities of the father or partner are very important and should not be trivialized. Fathers and partners strengthen and facilitate the process of co-creation by fostering comfortable and safe birthing practices that promote the development of a beautiful healthy baby. This chapter focuses on the roles and responsibilities of fathers and partners of the co-creation team.

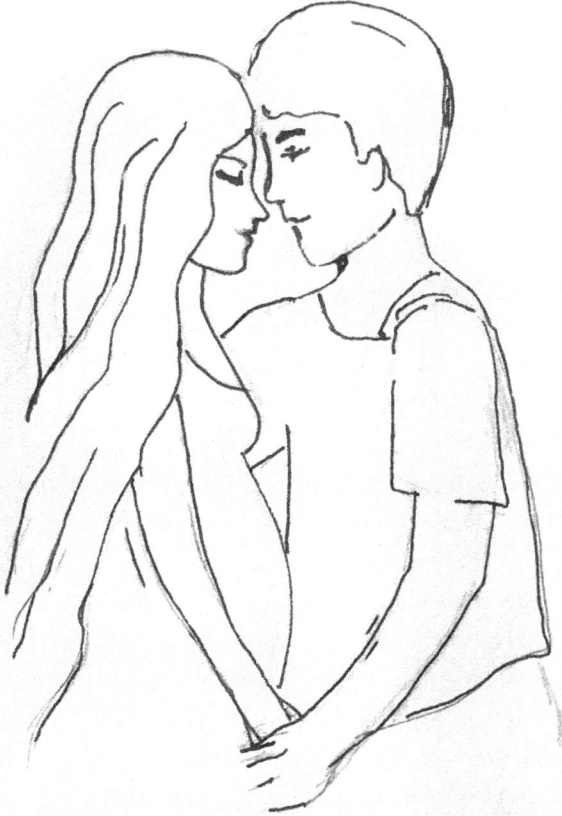

<u>Tips for Fathers and Partners during pregnancy:</u>

First of all, expect to experience a huge mix of emotions on hearing of the pregnancy. The more you think of it the more ambivalent your feelings may become. That's quite normal. While you are feeling ecstatic and excited at the news, you may also begin to feel anxiety about such things as:

- Financial Costs
- Your ability to be a good parent
- Your lack of knowledge about pregnancy
- Your changing roles and responsibilities
- Housing accommodation
- Loss of attention and constant companionship
- Changing sexual drive

Here is what you can do about these concerns:

1. COMMUNICATE, COMMUNICATE, COMMUNICATE

A. Accept, acknowledge, and express ambivalent feelings and thoughts without harsh self-judgment. The chances are that the mother-to-be may also be experiencing her own assortment of ambivalent feelings. Share your thoughts, dreams, hopes, fears, and anxieties with regard to having a child. Speak sincerely and lovingly, and listen attentively and compassionately. This is the time for deeper personal sharing. Then you can plan and work together to deal with any troubling issues. You can get help from a third party (friend, counselor, pastor, therapist, psychologist) if there are unresolved, deeper emotional issues that call for resolution and healing. Unresolved issues will come to the surface again and again until they are sufficiently addressed.

B. Set guidelines for effectively communicating with each other. During this period of your life when you can expect so many changes, it is vital that communication be open, honest, and regular. Decide **when?** (every evening during or after dinner); **what?** (feelings, thoughts and activities); **how?** (honestly and sensitively) **Why?** (bonding and supporting).

C Agree not to take occasional outbursts personally. Remember that a pregnant woman is experiencing hormonal and bodily changes that can easily trigger mood swings, changes in sexual interest, physical discomforts, and anxiety outbursts. You both may be experiencing frustrations that may cause an outburst.

D. Agree to make a greater effort to be more sensitive to each other—to be flexible, understanding, and to give unconditional love. Then you can tactfully remind each other of your mutual agreement to communicate and use some appropriate humor to diffuse any discord or conflict.

E Be constantly aware that all the emotions and thoughts of your pregnant partner are being transmitted to your unborn baby. So always try to help the mother-to-be to regain her balance quickly. An occasional outburst will not hurt your baby if it is corrected quickly, so do your best not to escalate anger or a heated argument or to allow negative feelings to simmer and create more toxic thoughts and emotions. That does more harm to you, your partner, and your unborn baby. Nobody wins in this scenario. You may think that this means backing down in an argument or not instantly addressing your own issues. Yes, you are right! In the interest of your spouse and your baby, you may need to do just that to prevent negative emotions from escalating. Then, you will have to find another more appropriate time to effectively deal with those troubling issues so that you can also enjoy peace of mind. In other words, one of your main roles will be to cultivate a happy, stable, emotional environment for yourself, for the mother-to-be, and for the growing fetus.

F. What can be a big challenge for a pregnant woman is her changing physical state. Do show appreciation and admiration for these changes. Strive to be sensitive to her feelings, and avoid making fun at her expense about her shape or walk. If she is concerned about returning to her prior shape, please reassure her that she can and will. Try to remove or reduce her anxieties. It requires real effort on everyone's part to patiently work through difficulties that will certainly arise. It is your love and commitment to each other and your growing baby that will help you to persevere to maintain a harmonious relationship.

G. It is important to discuss and appreciate the sexuality of childbirth. This will help you both to maintain a positive attitude towards birthing which involves the private sexual organs. It will also help the mother to surrender totally to the birthing process without sexual inhibitions.

2.   BE KNOWLEDGEABLE ABOUT THE PROCESS

A. To participate fully in this experience you need to gather information that will give you a comprehensive understanding of the whole process of pregnancy, birthing, and parenting. You may choose to begin by reading all of this book. There are many other books that you can also read. Refer to the bibliography, check out the internet and libraries, and watch films on this subject. Learn as much as you can. Then you and the mother-to-be can both share and discuss this information and be better able to make informed choices about what options would be best for you and your baby.

B. Accompany the mother-to-be to her prenatal visits, be it to the obstetrician, midwife, or birthing center. Demonstrate your role as a positive active member of the team. You will be respected for showing sensitive, appropriate support. Attend prenatal classes together and ask for answers to any questions that are relevant to you.

3.   ADOPT A HEALTHY LIFESTYLE

Use this experience as an opportunity to establish a healthy lifestyle.

A. NUTRITION
You can support each other by both eating a balanced, nutritious diet. This will help you, the mother to be and your baby to get the nutrients needed for healthy growth. If you eat right, then you will make it easier for her to eat right also.

B. EXERCISE, REST AND RELAXATION
There are many exercises that you can do together such as walking, swimming, and deep abdominal breathing. This can also

serve as quality and fun time with each other. Encourage her to do the ones that are specifically for pregnancy such as squatting and yoga. Stress and overtiredness can be harmful to both mother and baby at this time. So assist her with household chores and ensure that she gets time for rest and relaxation.

4.   MENTAL AND EMOTIONAL DEVELOPMENT

There are a number of exercises described in the mental and emotional chapters of this book that anyone can use for personal self-development. Please try them by yourself, or better yet with your partner. They will provide you with skills that will be beneficial in all areas of your life. Practice them all. You will be pleased with the improvement that you will experience in your mental and emotional functioning and in your overall performance. Encourage the mother-to-be to diligently practice these exercises so that she can strengthen her personal power and be the Birthing Goddess that she is meant to be. Working together on these exercises will help to build greater sensitivity between you.

5.   SPIRITUAL BONDING

This is a good time to acknowledge and strengthen your connection with your Divine Creator. The miracle of the birth of your baby will certainly touch your soul. Pray with gratitude and meditate together. Expectant couples who pray and meditate together reinforce their love and commitment to each other and their baby. This becomes a totally enriching experience for you both.

6.   FOSTER A DIRECT COMMUNICATION WITH YOUR BABY

- Talk, whisper lovingly, and sing to your baby. Do this often so that your baby recognizes your voice.
- Respond to baby's movement by gently tapping or caressing your partner's belly.
- Listen to your baby's heartbeat when you accompany your partner for checkups.

- Transmit positive, cheerful thoughts to your baby while you are in a meditative state. This has a profound effect on you and your baby.

Tips for Fathers and Partners during Birthing:

The big day has arrived! Regular surges have begun.

You have already mentally rehearsed what you have to do and all the preparation is in place. Now, take a deep breath, relax, and try to move as calmly and confidently as you can. Remember your role and responsibilities as stage manager of the production and protector of your wife, providing security, emotional stability and balance.

- Notify the other members of the birthing team —doula, midwife, or obstetrician. If you want to record the birth in pictures then engage a trusted family member or friend to be the photographer. Please do not try to play that role also. You have other more critical responsibilities at this time.
- Ensure that the environment meets the needs of the Birthing Goddess. In the early stages, allow her to rest and relax in comfort. Check her birthing wish list, if necessary. Arrange lighting, music, aromas, heating, water, juice—whatever she may need. Have the birth ball nearby and a warm bathtub available. If she wishes physical movement, assist or accompany her while walking in the garden, squatting, or sitting on the birthball.
- Be totally available to the birthing mother and your baby. Time her surges. If the birthing is going to take place at a birthing center or in a hospital, then make sure you leave on time to get there as you planned. If the birthing is taking place at home, then relax and do your part and allow the other members of the birthing team to do their part. Keep reminding yourself that you are the guardian of the birthplace. Be sufficiently assertive with visitors, medical staff, or birthing companions to ensure that the star of the show, your Birthing Goddess keeps her focus on her role. As the surges get stronger, continue to be sensitive, tactful, assertive

and gracious to your Birthing Goddess. Remember you know her best, so be alert to her cues. She may wish to be caressed, gently massaged, or to have sexual contact.

- Keep a respectful silence. Between contractions she may appear to be in a trance-like state. This is normal. The secretion of birthing hormones promotes a shift to an introspective state where her intuitive right brain and subconscious mind takes over. Don't try to initiate a conversation at this time. Watch for her nonverbal signals (that you may have agreed upon before), such as finger or hand signals for 'yes', 'no', 'come', 'stop' or 'go'.

  Try not to say words like 'relax' too often. That can be irritating and have the opposite effect.

- Speak softly, slowly, simply, and lovingly. You may say, *"You are progressing well"* or *"Feel yourself letting go as you breathe out."* During surges you can give gentle suggestions slowly and softly such as, *"As you breathe in feel the light energy flowing into your body, stretching and opening your cervix"*; *"As you breathe out see and feel your cervix softening and opening"*; *"Your birthing muscles are working well"*; *"Our baby is moving down slowly and easily into your birth channel."* Take care that your suggestions are not excessive or sound like orders. Your Birthing Goddess needs very sensitive support at this time.

- Give her a light touch massage. Gently and slowly using your finger tips, stroke her arms, neck, shoulders, back, spine, and her legs. Use a circular pattern when stroking her stomach. This feather like massage is very relaxing and comforting and facilitates the birthing.

- Give realistic support. Try not to make unrealistic statements like "It will soon be over" when the expectant mother is only 3 or 4 centimeters dilated. Instead, encourage her by giving feedback on what you see: *"I see you breathing deeply and relaxing more,"* or you may relate what your health provider says: *"Your midwife says that your have dilated 4 centimeters and our baby is positioned for a normal birth."*

- Communicate non-verbally. Look lovingly and tenderly into her eyes. Keep connected by touch: gently stroke her, hold her hand, kiss her, play with her hair, whatever she will appreciate. Transmit positive thoughts to her: words of encouragement, a prayer, a love song.

- Since each birthing is unique, be prepared for unexpected situations that can arise. Refer to your 'what if' plans to address such developments. If the birth is not going as planned, then you may be called upon to make informed medical decisions for the safety of mother and baby. Do so while maintaining your confidence and trusting in God's guidance. Relay this information to the mother-to-be in a tactful, positive, and loving manner. Assure her that everything will be all right. Keep affirming your love for her. Pray and visualize a safe and successful outcome and flow with the process.

- Welcome your baby as soon as he/she is birthed. Speak softly; say a prayer of gratitude while your baby is first caressed on the mother's chest.

- Do cut the umbilical cord and be aware of the significance of this act. You are now launching your baby into this world to continue his/her growth and journey as an individual.

- Reconnect with the mother. Hug, caress and kiss her tenderly. She may be exhausted physically and need to recuperate from the intensity of this experience. Imbue her with your energy. Snuggle and embrace her to keep her warm and comforted as you gently stroke her face and arms.

- Hold and gently stroke your baby as soon as you can. Look into the baby's eyes speaking lovingly and saying his/her name. Your baby will probably recognize your voice and you will be laying a foundation for a strong relationship between you and your child.

- Remain with your Birthing Goddess, even though the midwife or healthcare provider may be attending to her. She may experience labor shivers after the birth – so ensure that the room is warm and you have socks for her feet, if necessary. Pamper her, brush her hair, give her a drink, make her very comfortable. A Birthing Goddess deserves the best treatment.

SELF – CARE

Self-care is equally important if you wish to give good support through-out pregnancy and birthing. You too will need to plan and prepare your-self physically, mentally, emotionally and spiritually. Use this experience as an opportunity to develop and discover yourself more deeply as you participate more actively in co-creating your baby. Here are a few guide-lines to help you to cater to your own needs:

- Exercise regularly and find time for rest and relaxation with your partner.
- Find creative ways to balance your personal life and your work: delegate, arrange flexible working hours, prioritize frequently.
- Maintain your hobby if practical.
- Develop and utilize reliable and supportive relationships for yourself: best friend, family member, pastor, healthcare provider, or colleague. Share your concerns and anxieties with them, so that they can help you to address and resolve them. It is very important for you to maintain internal peace of mind and emotional stability at this time.
- Be aware of your stress level and take appropriate steps to prevent it from becoming *dis*tress. A high stress level will weaken your functioning in all areas of your life. Do make every effort to learn and to practice strategies to manage your stress. Remember too, that stress is infectious and can be easily transmitted from you to the mother-to-be and then to your baby.
- Practice mental rehearsals of the roles you have to play, especially during birthing. This will help you to clarify what you may be called upon to do and it will also help you to build stronger con-fidence in your capacity to give of your very best.
- The more involved you are throughout the pregnancy and birth-ing, the more fulfilling will be this experience for you.
- Remember always that you are an integral part of co-creation from the time of fertilization and conception.
- Your positive contribution to nurture the growth of that seed will help to ensure the total health and well-being of your baby.
- Do enjoy this Divine experience fully!

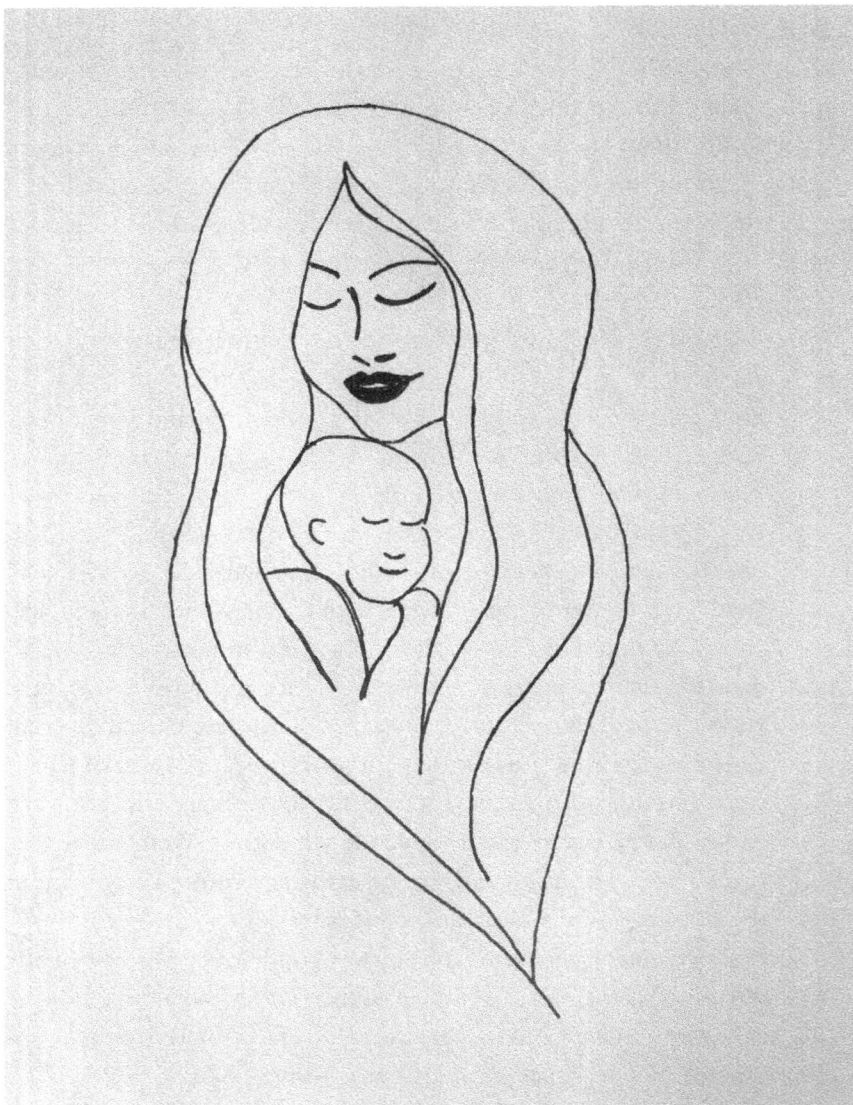

Chapter 8
The Birthing Goddess In Action

"The great end of life is not knowledge but Action"
Thomas Henry Huxley

Bringing a new life into this world is a sacred responsibility not to be taken lightly. Thorough preparation is necessary, so you must develop an effective plan of action that will prepare you totally for this major event.

Motherhood and pregnancy rearranges all our priorities. At this time your total well-being and that of your unborn baby are at the top of the list of priorities. The Action Plan that I suggest here is a holistic one. It integrates physical, mental, emotional, and spiritual activities into your daily life. This ensures that you are paying attention to the TOTAL YOU and giving the best to your baby's development. In this way you can maintain balance throughout your pregnancy, and achieve a high level of personal power that is necessary for a truly fulfilling natural birthing experience. Here is a Holistic Training Checklist and a suggested format for a Weekly Training Plan.

These are the exercises and activities that I have described in the previous chapters. Feel free to add others that are in-keeping with your goal for natural childbirth. Choose from the list what you can do for each week.

HOLISTIC TRAINING CHECKLIST

A. PHYSICAL PREPARATION

Breathing

- ☺ Slow deep abdominal breathing
- ☺ Surge and Expulsion breathing
- ☺ Alternate breathing
- ☺ Quantum touch breathing

Exercise

- ☺ Walking
- ☺ Squatting
- ☺ Stretching/yoga
- ☺ Swimming
- ☺ Dancing
- ☺ Pelvic floor exercises (kegels)
- ☺ Birth ball exercising

Rest and Relaxation

- ☺ Restful sleep
- ☺ Progressive relaxation
- ☺ Breathing relaxation with sound and imagery
- ☺ Massage and light – touch relaxation
- ☺ Meditation

Diet/Nutrition

- ☺ At least 8 glasses of water per day
- ☺ Lots of veggies
- ☺ High protein food
- ☺ Vitamins, minerals, and supplements
- ☺ A balanced Diet

Body Care

- ☺ Daily moisturizing
- ☺ Weekly massages
- ☺ Beautify, beautify, beautify
- ☺ Dressing attractively
- ☺ Regular visits to midwife/doctor/health care provider
- ☺ Perineal massage

B   MENTAL PREPARATION

Positive Thinking

- ☺ Controlling and cancelling negative thoughts
- ☺ Repeating affirmations daily
- ☺ Reading uplifting books with constructive information
- ☺ Being around positive people

Mental Exercises

- ☺ Focus of Attention Exercise
- ☺ Brain Fitness Exercise (3,2,1)
- ☺ Imaging & Visualization
    – Anchoring for confidence
    – Spiritual sanctuary
    – Bonding with your baby
    – Mental rehearsal

Self – Hypnotic Conditioning

- ☺ Relaxation
- ☺ Removing underlying fears
- ☺ Programming of positive suggestions
- ☺ Strengthening affirmations
- ☺ Deepening Techniques

C   EMOTIONAL PREPARATION

Purifying Negative Emotions

- ☺ Forgiving, Forgiving, Forgiving

- ☺ Practicing strategies to manage and cancel fear, anxiety, frustration, and anger.
- ☺ Resolving conflicts
- ☺ Managing stress
- ☺ Prayer and surrender to God

Nuturing Positive Feelings

- ☺ Keeping a gratitude journal
- ☺ Being a *"Good Finder"*
- ☺ Keeping a diary
- ☺ Sowing love – fostering positive, warm, loving relationships
- ☺ Reading uplifting books
- ☺ Anchoring your successes regularly
- ☺ Having fun—being frivolous!
- ☺ Celebrating yourself!

Creating a Positive Environment

- ☺ Developing a supportive team
- ☺ Surrounding yourself with your favorites: people, things, music, colors, aromas
- ☺ Watching happy movies
- ☺ Taking part in enjoyable fun-filled activities

D SPIRITUAL PREPARATION

Prayer

- ☺ Personal private prayer
- ☺ Family prayer
- ☺ Church and group prayer
- ☺ Reading religious and spiritual prayer books

Meditation

- ☺ Guided creative Meditation
- ☺ Hypno-meditation
- ☺ Surrendering to your Divine Creator

Support
- ☺ Maintaining spiritual friendships
- ☺ Listening to Joyful and spiritual music
- ☺ Watching happy and uplifting films
- ☺ Reading uplifting books

You can now use this Holistic Training Checklist to make your Weekly Training Plan.

There are some exercises that you may wish to include into your daily routine – such as meditation, abdominal breathing, squatting, and journaling. Then there are others that you may focus on as needed – such as anchoring, resolving conflicts, and gathering information.

You will notice that some activities can incorporate all or many aspects of your development.

- ➢ Meditation sessions can include: the mental focus exercise; deep breathing, self-hypnosis, rest & relaxation, affirmations, imagery, bonding with your baby, prayer, release of fears and negative emotions, peace and joy in your spiritual sanctuary, and surrender to God.
- ➢ Creative visualization can include: self-hypnosis, deep breathing, relaxation, positive programming, mental rehearsal and bonding with your baby.
- ➢ Walking can include: deep breathing, affirmations, prayers and contemplation.
- ➢ Squatting can include: mental rehearsal, reading, looking at TV, deep breathing, and affirmations.

Here is a format of a Weekly Training Plan that you can copy and use.

WEEKLY TRAINING PLAN "Happy Mother = Happy Baby"				
DAY	PHYSICAL	MENTAL	EMOTIONAL	SPIRITUAL
Monday				
Tuesday				
Wednesday				
Thursday				
Friday				
Saturday				
Sunday				

Keep your basic weekly training plan on the wall. Each week you can add to it or change it if necessary.

Try to put aside at least an hour a day to focus on your training (gym time!!). Throughout the day you can also take mini-breaks to stretch, do your kegels, squat, repeat your affirmations, deep breathe, pray, or connect with your baby. Many of these you can do while you are in your car.

You will be pleasantly surprised at how easily these activities will become part of your daily pattern of life – *your self-nurturing rituals.* You will be delighted with the positive changes that you will notice while engaging in this training.

So do CELEBRATE your progress and ENJOY!

BIRTH PLANS

1.   Birth Preferences Sheet

Whether you choose to birth your baby at home, in a birthing center, or in a hospital, it is always advisable to write out your detailed birthing preferences. This way your needs and wishes will be clearly understood by everyone involved in the birthing of your baby. Most birthing centers have their own birth preference forms that you can fill out beforehand.

2.   Roles and Expectations for Birthing Team Members

It is also a good idea to clarify the roles and your expectations of each member of your birthing party to avoid misunderstandings and to ensure that everyone is flexible and supportive throughout the process even if problems arise. Remember that you are a Birthing Goddess and that having a baby will be one of the most rewarding experiences in your life, so ensure you make the best choices for yourself and your baby.

3.   Birthing Bag

Have a birthing bag packed with whatever you may need during and right after birthing. Do this whether you are birthing at home or at another location. This way your birthing team will have these items readily available for you. Remember to pack your camera also. Your birthing center, hospital, midwife, or doula will be able to guide you on what you will need to pack.

4.   Breastfeeding

I do hope that you plan to breastfeed your baby. It's really the best way to go. The phenomenal benefits for you and your baby are well worth the time and effort you invest in breastfeeding. Seek the information and help you need from La Leche League or a Certified Lactation consultant. Getting off to a good start right after birthing can make it easier and more enjoyable for you.

5.   The "What If...Planner"

Be well prepared for any eventuality during birthing. Each birthing experience is unique. So keep in mind that there is always the possibility that the delivery may not go exactly as you planned. Be ready to make your adjustments calmly and confidently with the firm conviction that God is in control.

Go with an openness of mind to be sensitive to your body and do whatever your body needs to do. Set a realistic time limit and be receptive to medical intervention if needed. You may wish to spell it out clearly in your birth plan that you will have a cesarean only if other methods are not working and a life is in danger.

The "What If...Planner" will help you to think about and make conscious and informed choices that are in keeping with your wishes. Be sure to seek out all relevant information before making your decision. In other words, spend time before birthing to consider and discuss your options for "What if..." situations.

The What if...? Birthing Planner

What if...Birthing Planner (backup plans)	
Identify significantly disruptive "what if" situations which may occur and then determine the adjustments/strategies you wish to utilize.	
What if...	**Backup Plans**

<u>MY BIRTHING TEAM</u>

Clarifying Roles and Expectations:

1. Father/Partner:

2. Family Member:

3. Doula:

4. Midwife:

5.   **Obstetrician:**

6.   **Assistant/Nurse:**

7.   **Photographer/videographer:**

THE BIRTHING

Birthing usually takes place anywhere between two weeks before or after your due date and sometimes even out of that range .Your due date is simply an approximation. So be patient and be prepared:

- Your baby's accommodation and clothes are organized.
- You have your own birthing pack prepared – clothes, toiletries, music, etc.
- You have written out your birth plans, your 'what ifs' and clarified the roles and expectations of all members of your birthing team.
- You have done a good job of preparing yourself, and now you are ready to welcome your baby.

Ultimately, all your training is preparing you to do your best and let God do the rest. During birthing you are able to surrender to the Divine process. Genuine surrender does not mean giving up your skills and becoming passive. Surrender is handing over the controls to God *and trusting in your inner strength and personal power* to make the correct response to the miraculous process of birthing. This is the fulfillment of a Divine plan for you.

Here again, we experience the paradox of life – the coexistence of opposites. Precisely at the time that your whole system is subjected to a most intense strenuous activity, you are required to relax your body and mind. You are called upon to have greater control of your muscles and to relax them when necessary; to keep your focus on what is taking place within you and to surrender to the natural flow of the birthing process. The challenge here, as in all life, is to embrace both dimensions into one unified activity. This holistic program prepares you to meet this challenge. A well-prepared Birthing Goddess accepts and honors the entire birthing process, remaining calm and fully confident in the expertise of her birthing team, her own personal power, and in God's guidance.

You now have many options and techniques to utilize when you have begun your labor. During your mental rehearsal sessions you may have chosen the ones you intend to use during labor and birthing. When you have practiced them often and conscientiously, they become very effective for you during birthing. Utilize as many techniques and exercises as you can. ***The more choices you have, the more chances you have to succeed.***

Let us look now at what can take place during the birthing process. You may use the following as a **<u>Mental Rehearsal of the Birthing:</u>**

You are feeling progressive mild contractions or your amniotic membrane may have broken. These are signals of the onset of labor. Your birthing work has begun. You are well prepared and confident. You are experiencing regular surges. These surges may be anywhere between mild and intense and be 10 to 30 minutes apart. Each woman may have a different experience. This first stage of labor may also be short or long – a few hours or many hours.

You relax and flow with the process. If the surges began while you were sleeping, then you try to go back to sleep or rest for a while. You and your partner are probably feeling excited and raring to go. You turn that energy within.

You use slow, abdominal breathing and surge breathing. You go deep into a meditative state and into your inner sanctuary. You connect up with your baby and gently and lovingly urge your baby to position properly and play his/her part for easy and comfortable birthing. You visualize your birthing muscles relaxing and working harmoniously to open your birth channel.

You repeat your affirmations and give yourself powerful suggestions as you go to a deeper level of consciousness. You communicate with God throughout the process. You pray and surrender to His guidance. You conserve your energy and use it to facilitate nature's birthing mechanism. You allow yourself to flow in and out of the meditative state.

If you feel like walking, squatting, sitting on the birth ball, or any simple activity, you do so. A combination of rest and movement is working well at this stage. You drink liquids and eat lightly to keep yourself nourished.

Your birthing companion is playing his/her role in ensuring that the birthing environment meets your needs and that the other members of the birthing team are alerted and available. So you do not concern yourself with those responsibilities. You remember that you are a Birthing Goddess and the leading star of this show and you are well prepared to give your best performance.

Sometimes, your surges may slow down for awhile. You use that time to rest, relax and do your inner work. When your surges increase in intensity and duration and are occurring regularly every 4 to 5 minutes, you know that you are getting closer and closer to birthing. Your birthing companion will either drive you safely to the birthing location or alert the midwife to get to your home on time. Any relocation during birthing does not disrupt the process. You take it in your stride and keep your focus within as much as you can. When you resettle, you allow yourself to re-enter a meditative state to regain a deeper relaxation and inner centeredness. The body's natural birthing chemicals that relieve discomfort and speed up the surges are easily released to do the work that nature intended them to do at this time.

You welcome your surges as they become more intense and at shorter intervals. They are effectively dilating your cervix. You use the visualizations that you practiced and they work well for you now. You visualize your cervix opening like a flower coming into full bloom. You concentrate on directing your breath and your energy to your birthing muscles. Even though your surges are getting stronger and stronger, you are able to sustain a deep inner peace. You mentally repeat your affirmations and give yourself powerful positive suggestions.

You allow your instinct to guide you into whatever position or movement feels comfortable: sitting on the birthing ball, standing, lying, kneeling, squatting, on hands and knees, or rocking your body in any way. You do what's right for you and express yourself with sounds that come from your inner core. You allow your birth companion to cater to your needs – giving you a light-touch massage, maybe some water, or playing your favorite soothing music.

Your surges may also slow down and become less intense. You maintain your inner focus which enables you to calmly and serenely move in harmony with the natural birthing process. You keep your connection with your baby and your Divine Creator. As a Birthing Goddess, you allow the Divine to empower you every step of the way.

You know you are in the final stage when your cervix is fully dilated and you feel the urge to bear down. You change your breathing pattern now to expulsion breathing so that you can gently move your baby through your birth channel. You direct your breath downward and visualize your loving energy enfolding your baby and facilitating his birth. You push firmly and easily.

You can hear the encouragement, support, and prompts from your birthing team as you continue to focus on breathing your baby out into this world. You are a participant as well as a witness to this miracle of birth.

Your baby emerges from you and is placed immediately on your lower chest so that he/she continues to feel your warmth and comforting touch. You welcome and embrace your baby. You look into your baby's eyes and whisper loving words. You fully enjoy these first precious moments while sharing this magical time with your birthing companion. You experience indescribable feelings of relief, gratitude, fulfillment, and total joyfulness, and anchor these wonderful emotions in your mind so that you can relive them again and again.

Your spouse or birthing partner may wish to cut the umbilical cord and does so when the cord stops pulsating. Your baby suckles instinctively when put to your breast. This stimulation of your nipples helps your uterus to continue to surge so that the placenta is expelled quickly and easily. The midwife or doctor and assistants carry out their routine procedures while you, your partner, and baby continue bonding with unconditional love.

When you are ready, you then allow your baby to be 'cleaned up' and checked by your midwife or doctor. You also take this time to freshen up with the help of your partner or doula. Then you allow yourself to relax, rest, and be nurtured.

You go into a meditative state and thank your Divine Creator for empowering you to be your authentic self – a Birthing Goddess. You return to your private sanctuary, your own special place. You quietly celebrate your achievement and success. You allow yourself to float into the ethereal realms to enjoy the upliftment of a spiritual high. You have earned your glory. You feel wonderful. You remain in this state of ecstasy for as long as you need.

You then take your time and slowly and gently return to the full consciousness of your surroundings.

End of Mental Rehearsal.

You may use this mental rehearsal as often as you like and make whatever positive changes you may desire. By doing this Mental Rehearsal you are activating the energies of *The Law of Attraction* which affirms that what you think about you attract into your life.

Like a master gardener you have prepared the soil, planted the seed, fertilized, watered, weeded and mulched. You now have to wait patiently for nature to do the rest while still paying close attention to the process and praying that nature will support your efforts.

You are about to begin another fulfilling chapter in your life.

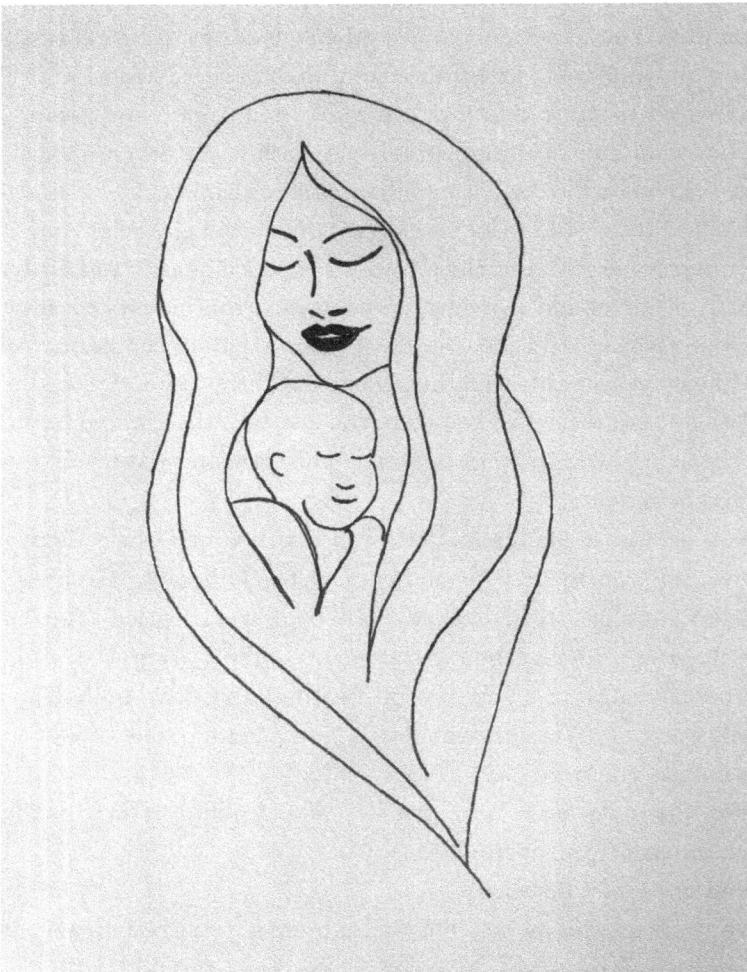

Chapter 9
A Higher Purpose

Your Contribution to Peace in our World

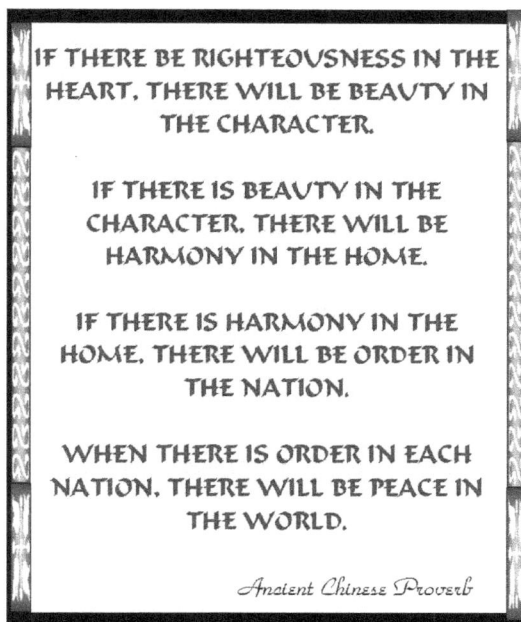

> IF THERE BE RIGHTEOUSNESS IN THE HEART, THERE WILL BE BEAUTY IN THE CHARACTER.
>
> IF THERE IS BEAUTY IN THE CHARACTER, THERE WILL BE HARMONY IN THE HOME.
>
> IF THERE IS HARMONY IN THE HOME, THERE WILL BE ORDER IN THE NATION.
>
> WHEN THERE IS ORDER IN EACH NATION, THERE WILL BE PEACE IN THE WORLD.
>
> *Ancient Chinese Proverb*

As a Birthing Goddess you accepted the responsibility to lay the foundation for the attitudes, values, beliefs, and behavior of your child from the time you conceived. You acknowledged that a pregnant woman's total state of consciousness affects the total state of consciousness of the baby in her womb. You made use of this significant window of opportunity to sow the seeds of peace, love and all that is positive into that new life. You were resolute in your desire to give your child the best possible start in life. You have succeeded. Commend yourself.

Every positive child is a valuable gift to the world and can produce a bountiful harvest of goodwill and joyfulness in the present and the future.

Each newborn brings hope for a better world:

Hope for peace within families, among communities, and between nations;

Hope for sharing love in its purest form;

Hope for more creative, constructive solutions to our man-made problems;

Hope for responsible management of our environment – our mother earth;

Hope for a safer, more joyful and fulfilling life;

This hope becomes a reality when these seeds of love and peace are nurtured by parents and the wider community. Our responsibility and influence does not end with birthing and parenting our biological children. It continues and extends to promoting peace and goodwill to all members of society. We can continue to sow positive seeds by purifying our thoughts and maintaining integrity in all our interactions.

This book focuses on the roles and responsibilities of biological parents. But the underlying philosophy applies to all other women and men who also can be empowered to rebirth themselves and influence and support others to rebirth themselves in a more positive way.

We can all contribute to a new generation of peaceful beings by beginning with ourselves. We do this by continuously strengthening our inner power through any balanced holistic development program similar to the one suggested in this book. Then we become empowered to be the best we can be and to do the best we can do. We are enabled to continue sowing positive seeds in all our interactions with others as we encourage each other to support and join with us in this noble endeavor.

The way toward a more peaceful world begins with each of us and then extends to our relationships with all others – with all children and all people in our own communities, in our nation, and in our world. Then we know that we are truly what our Divine Creator wants us to be – Birthing Goddesses and Godlike Beings, doing what we are sent to do – sowing positive seeds, co-creating new life, birthing and rebirthing in His image and Likeness.

Our world today may look dismal at times. But we as Birthing Goddesses along with our partners can commit ourselves to a higher purpose and a brighter future.

As civilization progresses, we all strive for improvement in every sphere of life: technology, systems, vehicles, nutrition. As Birthing Goddesses we must also play our part to improve the quality of our legacy as human beings. Marianne Williamson, in her book, *A Woman's Worth*, reminds us *"Women must remember the sacred nature of our Goddess self, the call to glory inherent in human incarnation. We are daughters of history and mothers to a new world. This is not the time to throw away our power. It is time to claim it in the name of love."*

**As Birthing Goddesses we have the power
to bring Peace to our world.**

Benediction

My wish:

May you enjoy a happy, healthy pregnancy.

May you achieve that ideal state of flow during birthing where you are deeply relaxed and highly focused, where everything flows smoothly and birthing feel soooo good, rewarding and blissful.

May this book inspire you and increase your passion to be the best you can be.

May we always remember **who we are:**

WE ARE BIRTHING GODDESSES.

May we remember **why we came:**

WE CAME TO CO-CREATE NEW LIFE *and to* CONTRIBUTE TO A MORE LOVING, HAPPIER *and* PEACEFUL WORLD.

May God be with us always.

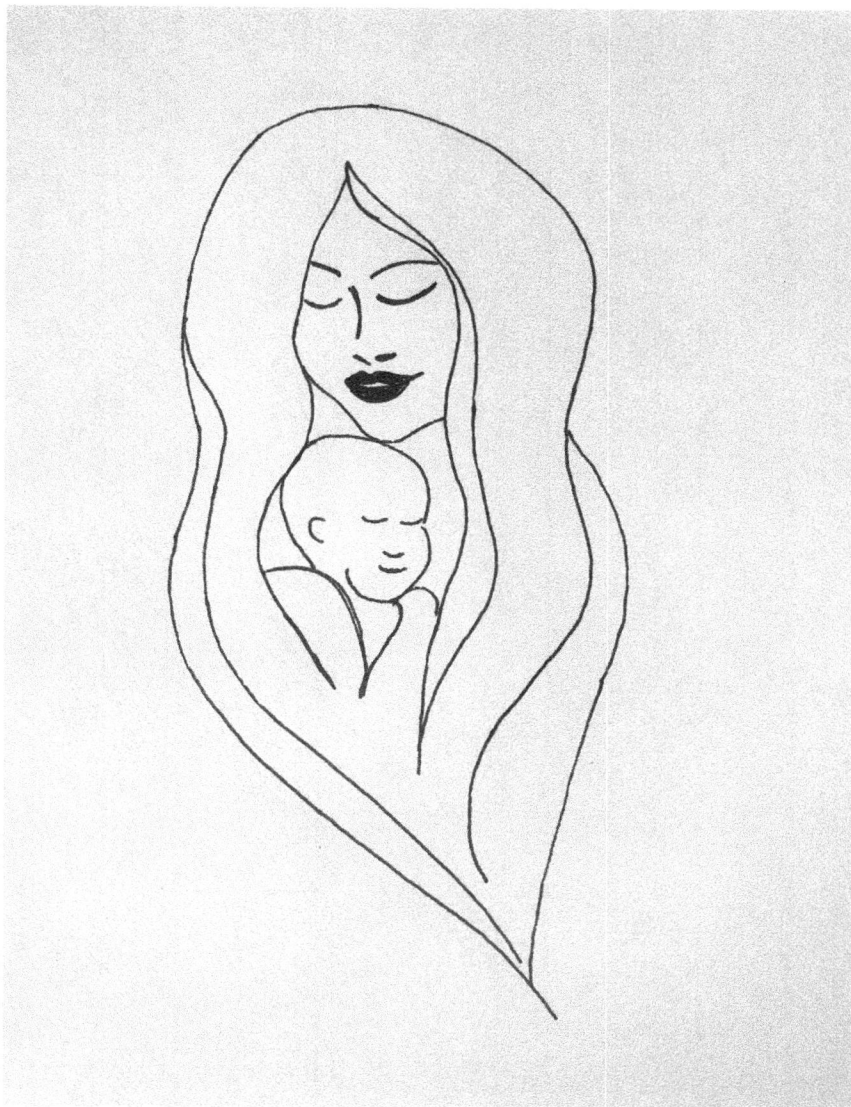

Bibliography

1. Childbirth without Fear – Dr. Grantly Dick-Read
2. Magical Beginnings, Enchanted Lives – Deepak Chopra
3. Hypnobirthing: The Mongan Method – Marie F. Mongan
4. Hypnosis for a Joyful Pregnancy & Pain-free Labour & Delivery – Winnifred Conkling
5. Painless Childbirth – Giuditta Tornetta
6. Painless Childbirth: The Lamaze Method – Fernand Lamaze
7. Creative Visualisation – Shakti Gawain
8. A Woman's Worth – Marianne Williamson
9. Preparing for Childbirth – Martin Rossman
10. Preparing for Childbirth: Guided Imagery Exercises (Audio CD) – Martin Rossman
11. Birthing from Within – Pam England & Rob Horowitz
12. Mind over Labor – Carl Jones
13. Meditations for Pregnancy – Michelle Le Claire
14. Visualizations for an Easier Childbirth – Carl Jones
15. Hypnotism & Meditation – Ormond McGill
16. Hypnotherapy – Dave Elman
17. Self-hypnosis – Charles Tebbetts
18. Emotional Intelligence – Daniel Goleman
19. Simple Abundance – Sarah Ban Breathnach
20. Illuminata – Marianne Williamson
21. Peace is Every step – Thich Nhat Hanh
22. Unlimited Power – Anthony Robbins
23. The Power of Positive Thinking – Norman Vincent Peale

24. The Power of Now – Eckhart Tolle
25. How to Stop Worrying and Start Living – Dale Carnegie
26. Use your Head – Tony Buzan
27. Quantum Touch – Richard Gordon
28. The Mental Game Plan – Bull, Albinson & Shambrook
29. Yoga for Women – Nancy Phelan & Michael Volin
30. The Molecules of Emotion – Candace Pert
31. The Power is Within You – Louise L. Hay
32. Meditations during Pregnancy – Beth Wilson Saavedra
33. Flow, The Psychology of Optimal Experience – Mihaly Csikszentmihalyi

www.ingramcontent.com/pod-product-compliance
Lightning Source LLC
Chambersburg PA
CBHW030014290326
41934CB00005B/336